ACUPUNCTURE POINTS HANDBOOK

Also by Deborah Bleecker

Virus Remedies Guidebook
Acupressure Made Simple
Tung Acupuncture Points
Acupuncture for Migraines
Shingles Relief
Natural Back Pain Solutions
Insomnia Relief

ACUPUNCTURE POINTS HANDBOOK

A Patient's Guide to the Locations and
Functions of Over
400
Acupuncture Points

Deborah Bleecker, LAc, MSOM

Disclaimer

This book contains the opinions and ideas of the author. It is intended to provide helpful and informative material on the subjects addressed. It is sold with the understanding that the author and publisher are not engaged in rendering medical, health, psychological or any other type of advice or services in the book. If the reader needs personal, medical, health, or other assistance or advice, a competent professional should be consulted.

The author and publisher disclaim any responsibility for any liability, loss or risk, either personal or otherwise that occurs as a consequence, directly or indirectly, of the use and application of the contents of this book.

Draycott Publishing, LLC

978-940146-20-1
12010

Contents

	Introduction	7
1	How Acupuncture Works	11
2	How to Locate Acupuncture Points	21
3	How to Do Acupressure Effectively	25
4	Ear Acupuncture – Auricular points	29

Acupuncture Meridians and Points

Bladder	35
Du or Governing Vessel	63
Gallbladder	77
Heart	99
Kidney	105
Large Intestine	121
Liver	135
Lung	145
Pericardium	155
Ren or Conception Vessel	163
Small Intestine	175
Spleen	185
Stomach	199
Triple Warmer or San Jiao	225
Extra Points	235
Resources	254
Index	255

It is health that is real wealth and not pieces of gold and silver.

Mahatma Gandhi

Introduction

This book is written for people who are interested in how acupuncture works. To understand acupuncture, you need to see how each point functions. Each acupuncture point has many functions. They all regulate the body, and restore normal function.

Although I have included information on Chinese medicine theory, it is not necessary that you understand Chinese medicine to benefit from this book. Each point is fully explained in both Chinese medicine theory, and Western medicine theory.

There are over 400 acupuncture points in this book. I could have easily made a book with 800. There are so many types of acupuncture, and so many ways to use the acupuncture points, that the topic is endless.

Meridian Images
The meridian images that are at the beginning of each meridian section include the point numbers. Due to the number of points in some areas, it is not always possible to number all the points on those meridian images. For more precise locations, see the individual points. I have also included images showing how to locate some of the more commonly used points.

Acupressure
If you would like to treat yourself with acupressure, I have included an explanation of how to treat yourself effectively. Please be aware that there is misinformation online. Always ask for the credentials of the person who is giving you advice. The problem is not that you would be harmed by advice that is not correct, but that you would conclude that acupressure does not work.

See a Licensed Acupuncturist, an LAc
If you would like to get acupuncture, it is best to find a Licensed Acupuncturist. In order to be licensed by the state, an acupuncturist must

have graduated from an acupuncture school, which is a graduate level program. A Licensed Acupuncturist has a degree in Oriental Medicine.

My degree is a Master of Science in Oriental Medicine, or MSOM. Other acupuncturists might have different types of degrees, but the goal is to find someone who studied Chinese medicine for three or four years in school. This will ensure you get the best care possible. Oriental medicine includes all aspects of Chinese medicine, such as Chinese herbal medicine, acupuncture, Gua Sha, cupping, moxibustion, and Tui Na, which is Chinese therapeutic massage.

Point Functions

I have chosen the most commonly used point functions and symptoms associated with each point. I compiled information from multiple sources. I have included how the points function in Chinese medicine terms if it is important to know. In most cases the functions are explained using modern medicine terminology.

Bulleted Lists for Major Acupuncture Points

The most commonly used acupuncture points are usually the points that have the most indications, or functions. I have indicated which points are commonly used by making the indication list a bulleted list.

The major points often have many functions and are much stronger than other points on the meridian. There are some points that are rarely used. They might be used to treat pain, by combining them with other points on the meridian, but they are less likely to be used to treat internal ailments.

Unbelievable Acupuncture

You might find it hard to believe that the points do what they are listed as doing. You are not alone. It is always surprising and even after 20 years of studying acupuncture, I continue to learn new points, and new ways to use the points I have known about for 20 years.

Chinese medicine is a very rich medicine. After over 2,000 years of use, it continues to grow. Although modern research has yet to be able to explain how acupuncture works, it has been shown to work as the primary form of medicine in China for thousands of years. It is able to heal things that modern medicine cannot, because it helps the body to heal itself. Acupuncture restores healthy function to the body. It helps your body to heal itself. If you have ever been healthy, your body knows how to heal itself. It just needs a stimulus to encourage it to heal.

Point Location

Most acupuncture points are located on both sides of the body. You can treat either side. Some points are located in the middle of the body, such as the Ren meridian, or the Du meridian, and there are special points that are treated on one side only.

Acupuncture during Pregnancy

There are points that are not to be used during pregnancy. You will find that different sources cite different points. The most commonly listed points to avoid during pregnancy are Spleen 6, Large Intestine 4, Ren 4, Bladder 31, 32, 33, 34, Gallbladder 21, and Bladder 60. These points are contraindicated during pregnancy, which means they should be avoided during pregnancy.

Although getting acupuncture during pregnancy will help the mother have a very calm baby, these points are typically avoided unless the mother is ready to give birth. In addition to using acupressure on Pericardium 6 to treat nausea during pregnancy, the point Bladder 67 is used to turn the baby when it is in a breech position.

Although some points should not be used during pregnancy, it is highly unlikely there would be a problem. In fact, some acupuncturists specialize in treating women during pregnancy, to relieve problems associated with pregnancy, or to relieve stress and improve energy levels. I do not recommend acupressure for pregnant women, without professional advice from an acupuncturist. Please see a Licensed Acupuncturist for help.

Naming of Meridians

Each meridian has a name. Some of the meridians are commonly referred to by their English names, and others by their Chinese names, such as the Ren meridian. The Ren meridian is also called the Conception Vessel. The Du meridian is also called the Governing Vessel. The meridian names tell you what organs they connect to, but that does not mean that is all they do. Each meridian is interconnected to other meridians. It is virtually impossible to treat one isolated ailment. Each point has so many functions, and the meridians are interconnected.

You will see several different names for a meridian. Other names include channel, and vessel. A meridian is a pathway in the body. When you stimulate an acupuncture point, it stimulates better circulation in the treated meridian, as well as the organs associated with it, and the meridians that are interconnected with it.

Notes for Acupuncturists

This book is not intended as a study guide for acupuncturists. It does not include the Chinese name for the points, the needle insertion depth, or the angle of insertion. The points are listed by number only, except for points that do not have a commonly used number, such as the extra points. The meridians are listed in alphabetical order, to make the points easier to find.

In this book there is a difference between Liver and liver. The capitalized word refers to the Chinese theory of the liver. In some cases, the theories merge, but I have attempted to capitalize the organ if the function is different from the Western function.

Chapter 1

How Acupuncture Works

It is not necessary for you to understand how acupuncture works to treat yourself with acupressure, or to learn what each point does, but the beauty of Chinese medicine is that it has its own system of diagnosis and treatment. For example, it is not necessary to know exactly what type of digestive problem you have, the points that regulate your digestion can be treated, and your body heals itself.

How Acupuncture Treats Pain
Pain is a large subject. There are so many ways that acupuncture can be used to relieve pain. The key thing to remember is that acupuncture of all types *restores normal blood flow to the area that hurts*. Pain is caused by a lack of healthy blood flow. After blood circulation is improved, the body can heal itself.

There are many options to treat pain. There are dozens of ways to treat each type of pain. Acupuncture also helps to break down scar tissue, and relax tight muscles. Nerve pain is relieved when acupuncture restores healthy circulation in the affected area.

When you get acupuncture to treat pain, in most cases other health issues can be treated at the same time. It is a truly holistic treatment. The whole body is treated. Acupuncture does not treat symptoms, it treats the underlying cause of the disease, and helps the body to completely resolve it.

Local or Distal?

Local points are located near the site of pain. *Distal* points are located further away. Back pain can be treated by choosing from about 100 acupuncture points. There are points on the hand, arm, leg, ear, and other places that relieve back pain. The type of pain you have determines which points will be most effective. There are several points on the hand that are very strong to relieve back pain. The style of your acupuncturist also determines which points are chosen.

To treat pain, acupuncturists determine which meridian is affected. When points on the affected meridian are stimulated, it restores normal circulation. We also treat not only the affected meridian, but points on the stronger meridians in the area. Distal acupuncture is done by treating points that balance the affected meridian. There are hundreds of ways to treat pain with acupuncture. For example, a basic treatment for arm pain might include Large Intestine 4, 11, and 15. These points strongly restore healthy circulation in the arm.

How Acupuncture Treats Emotions

In Chinese medicine, physical imbalances can lead to emotional imbalances. There is no separation of the mind and body. The mind affects the body, and vice versa. Treating the body with acupuncture and Chinese herbs is very beneficial to emotional health. You cannot be emotionally healthy if you are not physically healthy.

Emotions such as anxiety or stress are correlated to specific organ imbalances. Stress, for example, is related to your Liver. Anxiety is usually related to your Heart. Stress can be treated via the Liver meridian. Liver 2 and 3 are the most commonly used points for the Liver, although Spleen 6 also regulates the Liver. Anxiety and insomnia can be treated by regulating, and calming the Heart.

Points such as Pericardium 6, and Heart 7 are commonly used for anxiety and insomnia. There are often other imbalances that need to be treated. In fact, most people have multiple organ systems out of balance.

Chinese Medicine Diagnosis

A Chinese medicine diagnosis includes asking numerous questions. These questions tell us how your body is working. The questions might not seem to be related to your ailment, but they are in Chinese medicine. We will look at your tongue to see the general color and coating, as well as the shape. We take your pulse, which gives us more information about your health.

There are dozens of what we call *Organ Patterns* in Chinese medicine. You can have one, or you can have many of them. After a diagnosis has been made, acupuncture works to treat the underlying imbalances. Symptoms that seem to be unrelated to your health issue, can be very important in making your Chinese medicine diagnosis. The symptoms go away when the underlying imbalance is resolved.

Yin and Yang

You might have heard about Yin and Yang and wondered what they were. The theory behind them is pretty extensive, but I want you to have a basic idea of what they are, because certain acupuncture points treat the Yin, and some treat the Yang.

Think of Yang as hot, dry, and energy. It is related to the drive, and testosterone can be associated with it. As we age, our Kidneys decline. That causes a reduction in hormones. Yin is the cool, and moist. Yin correlates to estrogen. We all have Yin and Yang. Men have more Yang than women do. Children have the most Yang. They are bundles of energy. That is a very basic explanation, but I want things to be easy to understand.

Yin and Yang must be sufficient for the body to be healthy. There are many herbal tonics that are used in Chinese medicine to strengthen the Yin and Yang of the kidneys to improve health as you age.

Although there are dozens of organ patterns, I want to explain the most common ones. The organ patterns in this section are the most commonly

13

seen in clinic. If you understand how the organs function in Chinese medicine, it makes more sense how acupuncture can treat so many types of diseases.

Please remember that only *one* symptom is necessary to indicate that organ pattern is relevant for a health issue. In many cases, that is all someone will have, one symptom.

Kidney Organ Patterns

The most common imbalances in the Kidneys are a Yin or Yang deficiency. The kidneys are very important and treating the kidneys will resolve issues associated with aging. There are also anti-aging Chinese tonic herbs, which will improve energy levels, and treat disorders related to the Kidneys.

Kidney Yang Deficiency

Common symptoms of Kidney Yang deficiency include lower back pain, weak or painful knees, weak legs, feeling cold when others are comfortable, impotence, premature ejaculation, fatigue, frequent or profuse urination, apathy, swelling in the legs, and fertility problems. A Kidney Yang deficiency can often be correlated to a testosterone deficiency. In Chinese medicine theory, aging is associated with declining kidney energy. Ailments such as incontinence can often be resolved with acupuncture, and Chinese herbs.

Kidney Yin Deficiency

Common symptoms of a Kidney Yin deficiency are dizziness, tinnitus, poor memory, hearing issues or deafness, dry mouth at night, thirst, lower back pain, bone aches, insomnia, and night sweats. A Kidney Yin deficiency can often be correlated to an estrogen deficiency.

To treat Kidney imbalances, Kidney 3, 6, or 7 can be used. I like to combine all three points. Chinese herbs are often an important part of recovery from Kidney imbalances. Cordyceps is an example of a kidney tonic herb.

Spleen and Stomach Organ Patterns

The Spleen in Chinese medicine theory is completely different from the function in Western medicine. The Spleen in Chinese medicine is associated with digestion and energy production. The most common imbalance is Spleen Qi deficiency.

Spleen Qi Deficiency

A weak Spleen can cause a lack of appetite, abdominal bloating after eating, fatigue, pale complexion, weak arms and legs, loose stools. A spleen weakness can also cause excess fluid to be retained in the body. Stomach 36 is the strongest point to strengthen and regulate digestion, as well as improve energy levels. Weak digestion makes it more difficult to be completely healthy, as you do not get adequate nourishment from your food.

Stomach Fire

Stomach fire symptoms include a burning pain in the stomach area, thirst for cold drinks, constant hunger, bleeding gums, acid reflux, constipation, vomiting after eating, and bad breath. This pattern is not common, but it is similar to gastritis, which is an inflammation of the stomach.

Heart Organ Patterns

The Heart is affected by all emotions. Heart imbalances often cause anxiety, and insomnia. The Heart meridian is commonly used to treat Heart imbalances. Heart 5, 6, and 7 are often combined with Kidney points to treat the root imbalance. Stomach 36 can be used to improve energy levels, which impact the Heart.

Heart Qi Deficiency

When the energy of the Heart is weak, it can cause heart palpitations, shortness of breath on exertion, unusual sweating, pale face, and fatigue. Palpitations are when you feel your heart beating.

Heart Blood Deficiency

A deficiency of Heart blood can cause heart palpitations, dizziness, insomnia, poor memory, anxiety, being easily startled, a pale face and lips.

Heart Yin Deficiency

A Heart Yin deficiency can cause heart palpitations, insomnia, being easily startled, poor memory, anxiety, feeling emotionally restless, flushed face, feeling of heat in the evening, night sweats, dry mouth and throat, and five palm heat, which is when the palms of your hands and feet feel hot. This pattern is common in menopause.

Heart Fire

Heart fire causes heart palpitations, thirst, tongue ulcers, feeling agitated or restless, feeling hot, insomnia, facial redness, and a bitter taste in the mouth.

Lung Organ Patterns

The Lungs can be treated with acupuncture to resolve colds and flu, treat asthma, bronchitis, and any ailment associated with the lungs. Strong lungs ensure healthy energy levels.

Lung Qi Deficiency

A Lung Qi deficiency means the lung function is weak, which can cause shortness of breath, coughing, a weak voice, and a dislike of speaking. This can also be a side effect of a cold or flu. The coughing during a cold weakens the Lungs, which can cause a chronic weak cough. Some people never fully recover from a cold or flu, or bronchitis. The lungs remain weak. Herbs like cordyceps strengthen the lung energy, to help restore healthy lung function.

Phlegm Heat Obstructing the Lungs

Excess mucus in the lungs can cause a barking cough, which is a deep cough that sounds like a dog barking, profuse yellow mucus, shortness of breath, asthma, and a stuffy feeling in your chest. This correlates to bronchitis in some cases. The type of cough tells you what is causing it. A light cough is from weak lungs, a deep and barking cough is when there is too much mucus and inflammation in the lungs.

Wheezing is a common symptom of phlegm heat in the lungs. The lungs can be strengthened by herbs like Reishi mushroom, and cordyceps. Red Reishi mushroom is also a longevity tonic. Always take wheezing seriously, it can indicate a bacterial infection in the lungs, which should be treated urgently.

After you see your medical doctor for wheezing, your acupuncturist can help. There are herbal formulas that help to resolve the mucus, strengthen the lungs, and stop the wheezing. Stomach 40 is called the *Phlegm Point*, and it helps resolve mucus, and Lung 5 clears heat, or inflammation, in the lungs.

Herbs like Andrographis are used in Chinese medicine to treat bacterial infections. There is a famous herbal formula called *Chuan Xin Lian* that is very effective for infections. Chinese herbs must be taken very often, sometimes every two to three hours, but in my experience, infections can be resolved in a few days. I think Chinese herbs will more popular over time, as antibiotics have been overused and there are many strains of drug resistant bacteria. The herbs are broad spectrum, and typically have no side effects. I always refer patients to a medical doctor to treat infections. Infections can be life threatening.

Liver Organ Patterns
The Liver in Chinese medicine theory is very different from the modern medicine theory. The Liver is strongly affected by stress. Regular stress stagnates the Liver energy, which causes many ailments. Most people have some degree of Liver stagnation. Liver 2 treats Liver fire, Liver 3 treats most other Liver patterns. Acupuncture and Chinese herbal medicine are very effective to relieve stress. They help to relieve the accumulation of a lifetime of stress. Migraine headaches are often caused by Liver imbalances.

Liver Qi Stagnation

Liver Qi stagnation causes feeling irritated or stressed, sighing, hiccup, depression, nausea, vomiting, acid reflux, belching, difficulty swallowing, irregular periods, painful periods, breast distention, and lumps in the breast or under the arms.

One of the more interesting symptoms of Liver Qi stagnation is sighing. You will sometimes notice that someone is sighing a lot. That is the Liver trying to relieve stagnation.

A Chinese herbal formula called *Xiao Yao San*, or *Free and Easy Wanderer*, is very popular to treat stress. This formula is available over the counter, and it is one of the most balanced herbal formulas, which means most people can take it. If everyone took this formula, there would be a lot less stress and depression in the world. Stress affects your liver, which becomes imbalanced and that can lead to depression. It is also a common cause of infertility.

Liver Fire

Liver fire causes severe irritability, sudden outbursts of anger, tinnitus, headaches on the side of the head, dizziness, thirst, bitter taste, and a sudden flushed feeling when angry. Liver fire also causes facial sweating. When under stress, the heat flares up to the face, making it feel hot. Liver 2 is the best point for Liver fire.

Liver Blood Deficiency

Liver blood deficiency symptoms include blurred vision, floaters in the eyes, dizziness, insomnia, lack of menstruation, muscle cramps, brittle nails, and muscle weakness.

In Chinese medicine a blood deficiency is what causes eye floaters. If you have floaters, you can see black spots floating in front of your eyes if you look at a white wall. Many people have these and do not know it. They also rarely believe me when I tell them it can be fixed. It takes about a month. Blood tonic herbs need to be taken to restore healthy blood. I always have patients see an eye doctor to ensure there is no physical eye problem. A detached retina can also cause floaters.

Muscle cramps are also commonly seen with a blood deficiency. If there is not enough blood to keep the muscles nourished, they become tight and can cramp up. This can also cause neck and shoulder pain, as well as migraines.

Liver Fire is treated with Liver 2, and 3. A Liver blood deficiency would need to be treated by herbs, as well as points like Stomach 36 to improve energy production, and Spleen 6 to nourish the blood. Liver issues often cause menstrual problems, and infertility.

Dampness and Phlegm

It is a little difficult to explain the concept of dampness and phlegm in a short space. In Chinese medicine when the body accumulates too much fluid it is called dampness, which is called edema in Western medicine. In Chinese medicine theory dampness can be caused by either a weak Spleen, or weak Kidneys failing to remove the excess fluids. Chinese medicine is very effective to treat edema, it treats the root of the disorder by strengthening the organs responsible for fluid transportation in the body.

Phlegm is how Chinese medicine describes mucus. The mucus can be in your lungs during a cold or flu, and other ailments such as bronchitis. There is another type of phlegm that is not something you would see during a cold or flu. The word "phlegm" describes swellings in the body and imbalances that block organ function. Stomach 40 is the *Phlegm Point*. It treats all types of phlegm. Stomach 36 would also be included in your treatment, this point has dozens of functions.

These organ patterns are just the most commonly seen organ patterns in the clinic. This information is from Giovanni Maciocia's book *The Foundations of Chinese Medicine*. This is the textbook acupuncture students use their first year in school. It is an amazing book. If you would like to study Chinese medicine, I strongly recommend this book. There is no other book that really explains Chinese medicine like this book does. I am only giving a quick overview of common ailments, so the acupuncture points make more sense to you. Now, when your acupuncturist tells you that you have Liver fire, or Liver Qi stagnation, you will understand what he or she is talking about.

Chapter 2

How to Locate Acupuncture Points

Acupuncture points are located by using anatomical landmarks. For example, Pericardium 6 is located 2 cun from the wrist crease. You measure 2 cun by using your fingers. If you are treating someone who has smaller or larger fingers, you will use their measurements to locate the points. That means you would use their thumb size, rather than your own. You can also measure the point, and adjust the location slightly according to their measurements.

Many points are located using bony landmarks as a reference. The medial malleolus is an example of this. This is the round bone on the inside of the ankle. You place your fingers over the tip of the medial malleolus to locate the Kidney meridian points.

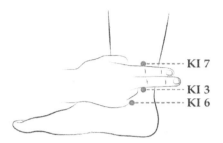

Kidney 3 is at the same level as the tip of the medial malleolus bone. Kidney 7 is 2 cun above Kidney 3, and Kidney 6 is below the medial malleolus.

Point Diameter

The size of each acupuncture point can be large. As long as you are inside the area, the point will be activated. The diameter can be the size of a nickel or quarter.

Cun Measurement

To locate acupuncture points, you need to have a way to measure distances on the body. That measurement unit is called a *cun*. That is the Chinese word for it. It is pronounced "Soon." Each cun is the size of your thumb knuckle. You will need to measure 1 cun, 1.5 cun, 2 cun, 3 cun, and 4 cun. If you are in doubt, you can always default to your thumb to do the measurement.

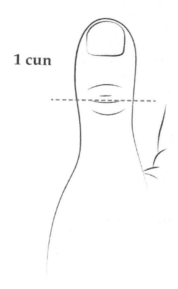

1 cun

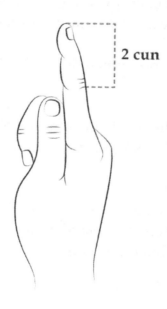

2 cun

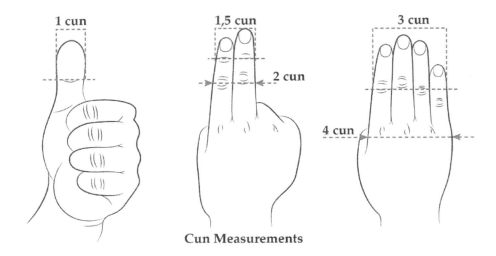

Cun Measurements

Anatomy Terms

The point locations in this book are explained as simply as possible. In some cases, I have used anatomy terms that might not be familiar to you. Rest assured that the images make the points easy to locate. The anatomy terms are used, but in most cases you can simply look at the image.

A few terms that you will see often include:

Medial Malleolus

This is the round bone on the inside of your ankle. This bone is used to locate points in the area, such as Kidney 3, 6, and 7, as well as Spleen 6.

Lateral Malleolus

This is the round bone on the outside of your ankle. This bone is used to locate points on the Bladder and Gallbladder meridians. It is also used as a point of measurement to find other points on the leg, such as Stomach 40.

Border of the Red and White Skin

This is a term that explains where the skin changes color. It is usually at the border of the sole of your foot, or the palm of your hand. It is not necessary to be able to see this to find the points to do acupressure.

Chapter 3

How to Do Acupressure Effectively

In order for acupressure to work, the point needs to be activated. With acupuncture, a needle is inserted into the point, which stimulates circulation in the point, which activates it. Acupuncture needles are tiny, about the size of a hair.

To activate the points using acupressure, there are several options.

- Pressing firmly with your fingers
- Using magnetic pellets on a piece of tape, which are applied to the acupuncture points and left on for a specific period of time, such as eight hours
- Using tiny seeds on a piece of tape that is applied to the ear. The seeds can be vaccaria seeds or other types of pellets such as ionic beads, or magnetic pellets
- Mini massager

The important thing to remember is that you must press firmly enough to activate the point. When you get acupuncture, the needles stay in place for about 30 minutes. While you relax, the needles have time to do their job. When doing acupressure, you will need to press firmly enough and long enough to stimulate the point. I would say five minutes per point is usually enough, but in some cases 10 minutes is necessary. It depends on which point is being treated, and how sick you are.

Treatment Frequency

Acupressure, like acupuncture, is a form of therapy. It is most effective if done daily. Every time you do acupuncture or acupressure, you are stimulating the body to function normally. If you only do it once a week, it will be less effective. Acupuncture and acupressure are both types of therapy, which means you need to do a *series* of treatments to get better.

Please do not expect one treatment of any sort to be all you need. I would plan on doing a series of four to eight treatments, and then decide if you need to continue. It can also be used for occasional problems such as nausea. The best point for nausea is Pericardium 6, which also treats insomnia.

Mini Massagers

Mini massagers are about 4 inches long, and they are used by some people for things other than acupressure. They are the perfect size to do acupressure. You can easily take them with you, and the tip is about half an inch in diameter, which makes it perfect to treat an acupuncture point. The best massagers for acupressure come with several different types of heads. The ones with the larger number of prongs seem to be the most effective for acupressure. These massagers cost about $10, and they can be bought online.

These massagers are also marketed to be used for scar treatments. Improving blood flow to a scar helps the body to break it down. Acupuncture is amazing to treat scars, as well as non-healing wounds, that are common in diabetics. Placing the needles around the wound improves blood flow, which helps the body to close the wound. A lack of healing is caused by a lack of circulation.

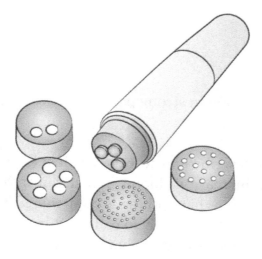

Magnetic Pellets

Magnetic pellets provide very strong stimulation to the points. I use the Helio brand of pellets, they come in a box of 100 pellets and each magnet is 800 gauss. Gauss is a measurement of how strong a magnet is. I have found these pellets to be very effective for insomnia, when placed on Pericardium 6. It is best to limit the time magnets are left on the body to eight hours. You might not feel them working, but they are very strong.

Acupressure Duration

The effects of acupressure are not usually felt immediately. It usually takes about an hour, although it depends on which point is being treated, and what results you are expecting. If you are doing acupressure on points like Large Intestine 11, to treat constipation, or Pericardium 6 to treat insomnia, you will usually see results in about an hour. If you do not see results, you can do acupressure again.

Getting the Qi

When you stimulate an acupuncture point, you are activating the point. Once the point has been activated, it starts to work. Acupuncturists call that "Getting the Qi," which is necessary for acupuncture or acupressure to work. The signs that you have activated a point include the following sensations in the area being treated:

- Itching
- Tingling
- Numbness
- Aching (more common in strong points like Stomach 36)
- Warmth

Sometimes you cannot describe how it feels, you just know something is going on, you feel the increase in blood flow. Even if you do not feel anything that does not mean that nothing is happening. If you have very low energy levels, you will be less likely to feel anything until your energy levels are built up, which usually takes about a month.

Ear Acupressure

Ear acupressure is another way to treat yourself. The ear is very sensitive to any type of stimulation. You can buy ear seeds online. There are several different types. The seeds are placed on a tiny square piece of tape. After applying the seeds to the ear, the tape will last a couple of days, depending on how often you shampoo, and how strong the tape is.

I like Sakamura ion pellets. They come in two types, the tape is either clear or flesh colored, and the pellets are either gold or silver. It is a matter of personal preference. I use clear tape with gold pellets. It is best to remove the pellets after two days and switch to the other ear.

Chapter 4

Ear Acupuncture or Acupressure

The ear is a microcosm of the whole body. That means the whole body is represented on the ear. The map of the ear shows the body represented as an upside down fetus. All ailments can be treated on the ear. The ear can be used to treat internal organ imbalances, pain, emotional issues, and to regulate the entire body.

The image below shows the inverted fetus. You will notice the head at the bottom of the image. The internal organs are located on the inner part of the ear, by the ear canal.

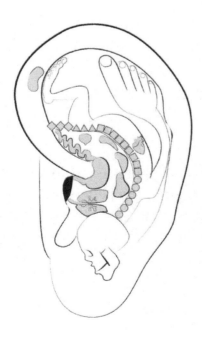

Some acupuncturists specialize in ear acupuncture. Many acupuncturists combine ear acupuncture with body acupuncture to get the benefits of both. Ear acupuncture and acupressure are especially useful to treat pain. Just locate the area on the ear that corresponds to the body part that is painful.

The ear points can be stimulated using tiny acupuncture needles, ear seeds that are made with vaccaria seeds, which are tiny black seeds that are placed on a small piece of tape. The seeds are placed on the ear and can be left on several days, they usually fall off within a few days. It is common to alternate ears, which means that for one treatment the right ear is treated, and the left ear is treated for the following visit.

Ear Seeds
The image below shows vaccaria seeds on little plastic flats, you just unpeel the piece of tape and place it on the ear. Using tweezers makes it easier.

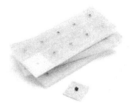

There are numerous types of small pellets typically used on the ear. Another type of ear pellet is Magrain Ion pellets from Sakamura. These are tiny beads, either gold or silver, attached to round pieces of tape. The beads are treated to provide stimulation that is not as strong as a magnet, but stronger than a vaccaria seed.

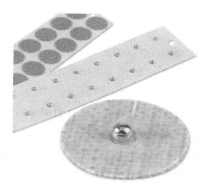

This image shows Sakamura Magrain Ion pellets on flesh colored tape. There are two options, clear tape, or flesh colored tape, and gold or silver pellets. Your acupuncturist will have a personal preference on which type of pellets are used.

Ear acupuncture is also used to help relieve drug addiction. Ear acupuncture relieves stress and can be used by non-acupuncturists to help in addiction protocols. The following image shows the NADA ear protocol used by addiction specialists. NADA stands for National Acupuncture Detoxification Association. There is special training offered for those interested in learning the protocol. For more information, please refer to www.acudetox.com.

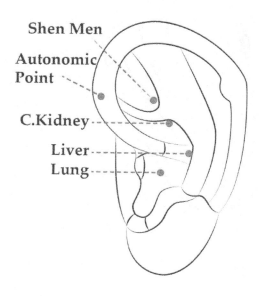

The following chart shows the spine represented on the ear. The points C1 to C7 represent the cervical, or neck vertebrae. I have found that treating these points on the ear with Sakamura pellets is as effective as any other type of neck treatment. Just place the pellets on the edge of the ear in the corresponding affected area and press firmly. When you press firmly, it will hurt a little. It will only hurt if there is a problem in that area. The points T1 to T 12 treat the thoracic, or upper back area. L1 to L5 are for the lumbar, or lower back area. S1 and 2 are for the sacrum, or tailbone.

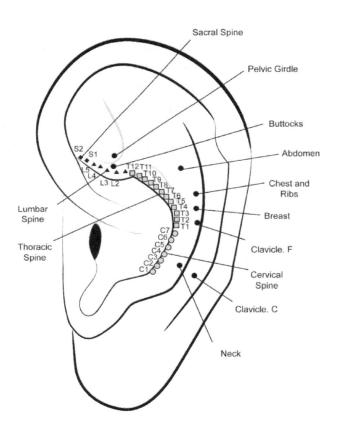

Commonly Used Ear Points

Shen Men

Shen Men is a master point. It calms the mind, relieves stress, pain, anxiety, insomnia, and it is used in combination with other points. The name means "Spirit Gate." It is one of the most commonly used points on the ear.

Point Zero

This point balances the body. It helps to regulate hormones, and calm the brain.

Tranquilizer Point

This point is also called the Relaxation Point, or Valium Analogue Point, by Terry Oleson. It is sedating, and relaxing and can be used to treat anxiety, high blood pressure, and chronic stress.

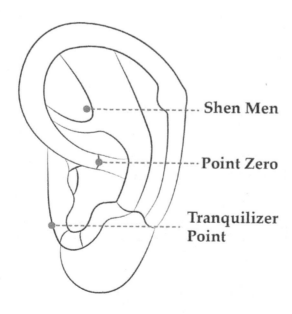

There are several systems of ear acupuncture. If you interested in further study, the book *Auriculotherapy Manual* by Terry Oleson, PhD, is a good choice.

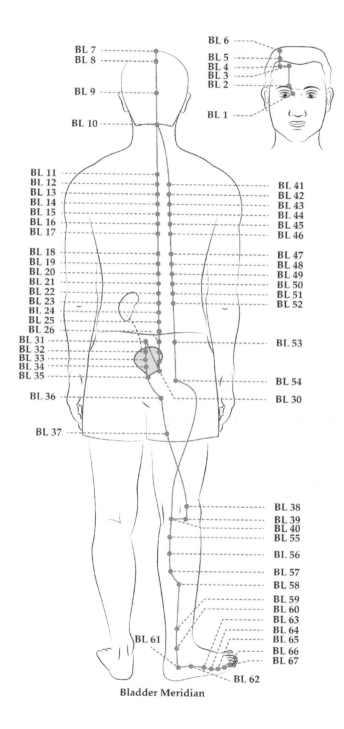

BL 7
BL 8
BL 9
BL 10

BL 6
BL 5
BL 4
BL 3
BL 2
BL 1

BL 11
BL 12
BL 13
BL 14
BL 15
BL 16
BL 17
BL 18
BL 19
BL 20
BL 21
BL 22
BL 23
BL 24
BL 25
BL 26
BL 31
BL 32
BL 33
BL 34
BL 35
BL 36
BL 37

BL 41
BL 42
BL 43
BL 44
BL 45
BL 46
BL 47
BL 48
BL 49
BL 50
BL 51
BL 52
BL 53
BL 54
BL 30

BL 38
BL 39
BL 40
BL 55
BL 56
BL 57
BL 58
BL 59
BL 60
BL 63
BL 64
BL 65
BL 66
BL 67

BL 61
BL 62

Bladder Meridian

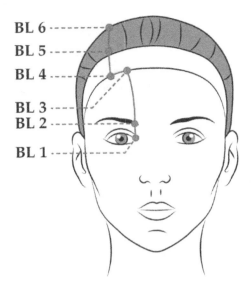

Bladder 1
Located .1 cun superior to the inner canthus of the eye.

Functions and Common Usage
Opens and brightens the eyes. Can be used for most types of eye diseases, including glaucoma, cataracts, optic nerve atrophy, color blindness, nearsightedness, eye swelling, eye pain, blurred vision, and sudden blindness. Bladder 1, like other points around the eye, stimulates healthy nerve function in the eye. Acupuncture restores nerve function and the body heals itself.

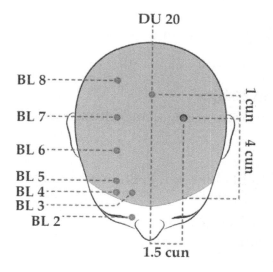

Bladder 2

On the medial, or inner, end of the eyebrow.

Functions and Common Usage

This point can be used for the same indications as Bladder 1, to treat all eye diseases. In addition to eye issues, it can be used to open the sinuses to treat allergies, and sinus congestion or pain.

Bladder 3

Located above the medial end of the eyebrow, .5 cun above the front hairline.

Functions and Common Usage

Clears the head to relieve headache, also treats sinus congestion.

Bladder 4

Located .5 cun above the front hairline, 1.5 cun from the midline.

Functions and Common Usage

Can be used for sinus congestion.

Bladder 5
Located 1.5 cun lateral to the midline, and .5 cun directly above Bladder 4.

Functions and Common Usage
Can be used for sinus congestion, vertigo, and blurred vision.

Bladder 6
Located 1.5 cun posterior to Bladder 5, 1.5 cun lateral to the midline.

Functions and Common Usage
Clears the sinuses to treat sinus blockage.

Bladder 7
Located 1.5 cun posterior to Bladder 6, 1.5 cun lateral to the midline.

Functions and Common Usage
Regulates the nose to treat sinus congestion, loss of sense of smell, inflamed sinuses, and headache.

Bladder 8
Located 1.5 cun posterior to Bladder 7, 1.5 cun lateral to the midline.

Functions and Common Usage
Treats the eyes and nose. Can be used to treat sinus congestion, and blurred vision.

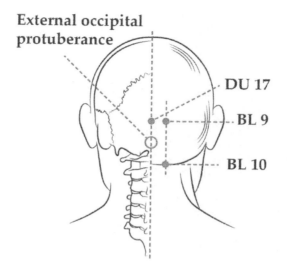

Bladder 9

Located 1.3 cun lateral to Du 17 at the midline, on the lateral side of the superior border of the external occipital protuberance, which is the bony knot on the back of your head.

Functions and Common Usage

Treats the nose and eyes. Can be used for sinus congestion, and eye pain.

Bladder 10

Located 1.3 cun lateral to Du 15, in the depression on the lateral side of the trapezius muscle.

Functions and Common Usage

Opens the nose, treats eye pain, neck stiffness, headache at the base of the head, and whiplash.

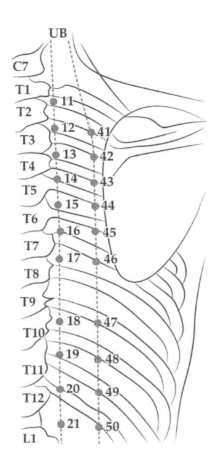

Bladder 11
Located 1.5 cun lateral to the midline, at the level of the lower border of the first thoracic vertebra.

Functions and Common Usage
Regulates the lungs, expands and relaxes the chest to treat ailments such as pneumonia, bronchitis, cough, cold and flu, and pleurisy. It also treats bone disorders by strengthening the bones and relaxing the tendons. Treats spine stiffness, joint deformity, and stiff neck.

Bladder 12
Located 1.5 cun lateral to the midline, at the lower border of the second thoracic vertebra.

Functions and Common Usage

Regulates the Lungs, which could be used to treat colds and flu, pneumonia, bronchitis, pleurisy, and whooping cough. It also opens the sinuses to treat sinus congestion, and discharge.

Bladder Shu Points

Bladder 13 begins the series of points called "Back Shu" points. This can be translated as "Associated" points. Each point corresponds to a specific organ. They can be used to treat chronic health conditions of the associated organ. For example, the Lung Associated point is Bladder 13, which means that point is used to treat Lung disorders. Bladder 14 treats the Pericardium, Bladder 15 treats the Heart, etc. Acupuncturists call these points Back Shu points, but I am avoiding using Chinese Pin Yin, because I want to use a more familiar term. I will refer to all "Shu" points as "Associated Point" for ease of use.

Bladder 13

Located 1.5 cun lateral to Du 12, at the lower border of the third thoracic vertebra.

Functions and Common Usage

Lung Associated Point. Bladder 13 regulates and tonifies the Lungs. Can be used to treat difficult breathing, cold and flu, excess mucus in the lungs, asthma, bronchitis, and cough.

Bladder 14

Located 1.5 cun lateral to the midline, at the lower border of the fourth thoracic vertebra.

Functions and Common Usage

Pericardium Associated Point. It regulates and strengthens the Heart, improves circulation in the chest, and it can be used to treat chest pain, palpitations, intercostal neuralgia (rib pain), and coughing.

Bladder 15

Located 1.5 cun lateral to the midline, at the lower border of the spinous process of the fifth thoracic vertebra.

Functions and Common Usage

Heart Associated Point. It regulates and strengthens the Heart, clears Heart Fire, restores normal circulation in the chest, and calms the mind. It can be used to treat cough, chest pain, insomnia, anxiety, palpitations, and coughing blood.

Bladder 16

Located 1.5 cun lateral to the midline, at the level of the lower border of the spinous process of the sixth thoracic vertebra.

Functions and Common Usage

Governing vessel (Du meridian) Associated Point. According to some sources the most common modern usage is to treat skin diseases such as psoriasis, and itching. Another source indicates it restores circulation in the chest and can be used to treat pericarditis, endocarditis, diaphragm spasms, and chest pain.

Bladder 17
Located 1.5 cun lateral to the midline, at the level of the lower border of the spinous process of the seventh thoracic vertebra.

Functions and Common Usage
Diaphragm Associated Point. Regulates the blood, moves stagnant blood, and clears blood heat. Bladder 17 regulates the diaphragm to treat hiatal hernia, esophageal constriction, and acid reflux.

Bladder 18
Located 1.5 cun lateral to the midline, at the level of the lower border of the spinous process of the ninth thoracic vertebra.

Functions and Common Usage
Liver Associated Point. Bladder 18 regulates the Liver and Gallbladder. It treats digestive issues such as jaundice, and pancreatitis. It brightens the eyes, it can be used to treat eye disorders such as blurred vision, optic nerve atrophy, and night blindness.

Bladder 19
Located 1.5 cun lateral to the midline, at the level of the lower border of the spinous process of the tenth thoracic vertebra.

Functions and Common Usage
Gallbladder Associated Point. Bladder 19 regulates the Liver and Gallbladder. It could be used to treat jaundice, vomiting, and pancreatitis. It clears damp heat from the Liver and Gallbladder, which can be translated as treating jaundice, or other Liver or Gallbladder disorders associated with inflammation.

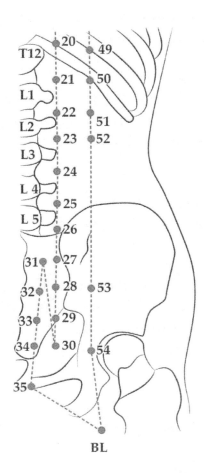

Bladder 20
Located 1.5 cun lateral to the midline, at the level of the lower border of the spinous process of the eleventh thoracic vertebra.

Functions and Common Usage
Spleen Associated Point. Bladder 20 regulates and strengthens the Spleen (digestion), improves digestion, and energy levels.

Bladder 21

Located 1.5 cun lateral to the midline, at the level of the lower border of the spinous process of the twelfth thoracic vertebra.

Functions and Common Usage

Stomach Associated Point. Bladder 21 tonifies the Spleen, raises Spleen Qi, and holds the blood. Translation: Improves digestion, regulates digestion, treats edema, and fatigue. It can be used to treat digestive issues such as diarrhea, nausea, and pain in the stomach area. The expression "holds the blood" means that it regulates the blood.

Bladder 22

Located 1.5 cun lateral to the midline, at the level of the lower border of the spinous process of the first lumbar vertebra.

Functions and Common Usage

Triple Burner or San Jiao Associated Point. Bladder 22 regulates the Triple Burner, and strengthens the Kidneys. Can be used to treat edema, nephritis, digestive issues, and to activate the bladder to expel urinary tract or kidney stones. The Triple Burner is an ancient concept that describes the flow of energy in the body. There is an Upper, Middle, and Lower Burner, each corresponding to specific organs.

Bladder 23

Located 1.5 cun lateral to the midline, at the level of the lower border of the spinous process of the second lumbar vertebra.

Functions and Common Usage

Kidney Associated Point. Strengthens the kidneys, and tonifies all aspects of the kidneys. Regulates urination, which can promote urination in cases of painful urinary problems. Treats urinary incontinence, edema, and chronic nephritis. Treats the ears and brightens the eyes, could be used to treat hearing problems, tinnitus, deafness, and blurred vision. Strengthens the lower back to treat back pain caused by Kidney deficiency.

Bladder 24

Located 1.5 cun lateral to the midline, at the level of the lower border of the spinous process of the third lumbar vertebra.

Functions and Common Usage

Sea of Qi Associated Point. Improves energy levels, and strengthens the lower back. Can be used to treat lower back pain.

Bladder 25

Located 1.5 cun lateral to the midline, at the level of the lower border of the spinous process of the fourth lumbar vertebra.

Functions and Common Usage

Large Intestine Associated Point. It regulates the intestines, and strengthens the lower back and knees. It can be used to treat constipation, rectal prolapse, and hemorrhoids.

Bladder 26

Located 1.5 cun lateral to the midline, at the level of the lower border of the spinous process of the fifth lumbar vertebra.

Functions and Common Usage

Gate of Origin Associated Point. Bladder 26 strengthens the lower back. It can be used to treat lower back pain.

Bladder 27

Located 1.5 cun lateral to the midline, at the level of the first posterior sacral foramen. Translation: The sacral foramen are holes in the sacrum, which is also called the tailbone.

Functions and Common Usage

Small Intestine Associated Point. Regulates the intestines and bladder. It can be used to treat peritonitis, and colic. It can also be used to treat damp heat syndromes causing difficult urination. Damp heat could be seen as a type of inflammation, there is too much heat, or inflammation, in the body.

Bladder 28
Located 1.5 cun lateral to the midline, at the level of the second posterior sacral foramen.

Functions and Common Usage
Bladder Associated Point. Bladder 28 regulates the bladder. It can be used to treat painful urinary dysfunction, prostatitis, and lower back pain. It strengthens the lower back.

Bladder 29
Located 1.5 cun lateral to the midline, at the level of the third posterior sacral foramen.

Functions and Common Usage
Mid-Spine Associated Point. It is also translated as Central Spine Hollow. It strengthens the lower back to treat spine stiffness, and pain.

Bladder 30
Located 1.5 cun lateral to the midline, at the level of the fourth posterior sacral foramen.

Functions and Common Usage
White Ring Associated Point. The translation of this refers to the anus. It can be used to treat lower back pain, and urinary incontinence due to paralysis. Although infrequently used, it could be used to treat back pain.

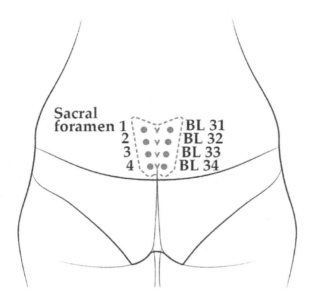

Bladder 31

In the first posterior sacral foramen, which are holes in your tailbone.

Functions and Common Usage

Bladder 31, 32, 33, 34 are called the Eight Foramen points. They are often used together to treat lower back pain, sacrum, and coccyx, or tailbone pain. Although there are about 100 points on the body that can be used to treat back pain, these points are very effective to restore blood flow and relax the muscles in the back.

Bladder 32
In the second posterior sacral foramen.

Functions and Common Usage
See above.

Bladder 33
In the third posterior sacral foramen.

Functions and Common Usage
See above.

Bladder 34
In the fourth posterior sacral foramen.

Functions and Common Usage
See above.

Bladder 35
On both sides of the tip of the coccyx, or tailbone, .5 cun lateral to the midline. Notice how the Bladder meridian splits at this point and goes down the leg to the end of the little toe. There are two Bladder meridian lines on the back, the inner and the outer line.

Functions and Common Usage
Can be used to treat tailbone pain, although there are many other points to treat this that are more easily accessed.

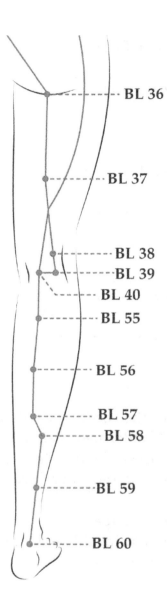

BL 36

BL 37

BL 38
BL 39
BL 40
BL 55

BL 56

BL 57
BL 58

BL 59

BL 60

Bladder 36

In the center of the gluteal fold. Translation: the gluteal fold is located beneath the buttocks.

Functions and Common Usage

Bladder 36 strengthens the lower back, and can be used to relieve pain in the lower back. It is also listed as treating hemorrhoids.

Bladder 37

Located 6 cun below Bladder 36, on the line joining Bladder 36 and 40.

Functions and Common Usage

Bladder 37 strengthens the lower back. It can be used to relieve lower back pain, sciatica, and atrophy of the leg.

Bladder 38

Located 1 cun above Bladder 39, on the medial side of the biceps femoris tendon. Located with a flexed knee.

Functions and Common Usage

Relaxes the tendons, and relieves lower back pain.

Bladder 39

Lateral to Bladder 40, on the medial border of the biceps femoris tendon.

Functions and Common Usage

Regulates the Triple Burner to treat abdominal distension. Could be used to treat knee pain.

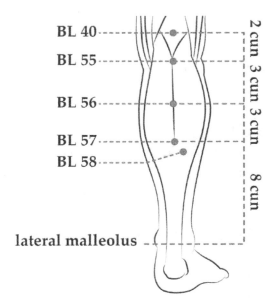

Bladder 40

Located at the midpoint of the popliteal fossa. Translation: located behind the knee, at roughly the midpoint.

Functions and Common Usage

Strengthens the lower back to relieve back pain. It relaxes the tendons, and can be used to treat back pain that causes stiffness, and the inability to stand up straight.

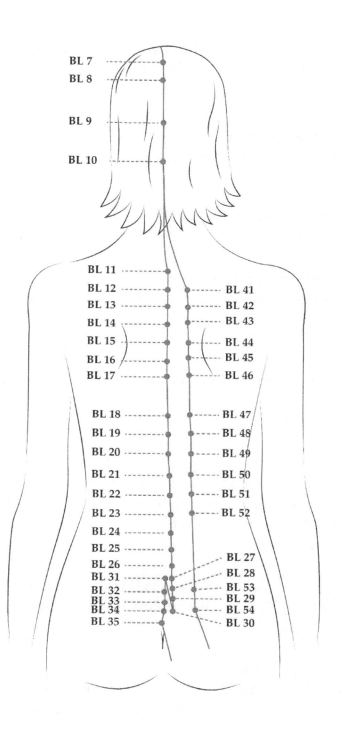

BL 7
BL 8
BL 9
BL 10
BL 11
BL 12
BL 13
BL 14
BL 15
BL 16
BL 17
BL 18
BL 19
BL 20
BL 21
BL 22
BL 23
BL 24
BL 25
BL 26
BL 31
BL 32
BL 33
BL 34
BL 35
BL 41
BL 42
BL 43
BL 44
BL 45
BL 46
BL 47
BL 48
BL 49
BL 50
BL 51
BL 52
BL 27
BL 28
BL 53
BL 29
BL 54
BL 30

53

Bladder 41
Located 3 cun lateral to the midline, at the level of the lower border of the spinous process of the second thoracic vertebra, on the spinal border of the scapula.

Functions and Common Usage
Can be used to treat back pain, or shoulder pain.

Bladder 42
Located 3 cun lateral to the midline, at the level of the lower border of the spinous process of the third thoracic vertebra.

Functions and Common Usage
Strengthens the lungs. It can be used to treat difficult breathing and cough.

Bladder 43
Located 3 cun lateral to the midline, at the level of the lower border of the spinous process of the fourth thoracic vertebra, on the spinal border of the scapula.

Functions and Common Usage
Strengthens the lungs, and kidneys. Can be used to treat lung issues such as bronchitis, asthma, and tuberculosis. These ailments would commonly be treated with Chinese herbal medicine.

Bladder 44
Located 3 cun lateral to Du 11, at the level of the lower border of the spinous process of the fifth thoracic vertebra, on the spinal border of the scapula.

Functions and Common Usage
Regulates the heart, and improves circulation in the chest. Can be used to treat cough, or difficult breathing. Points on the Lung meridian would be more commonly used over points on the back in many cases.

Bladder 45

Located 3 cun lateral to Du 10, at the level of the lower border of the spinous process of the sixth thoracic vertebra.

Functions and Common Usage

Regulates the lungs to treat cough, and difficult breathing. It treats shoulder, scapula, and back pain.

Bladder 46

Located 3 cun lateral to Du 9, at the level of the lower border of the spinous process of the seventh thoracic vertebra, near the lower border of the scapula.

Functions and Common Usage

Regulates the diaphragm, which can be used to treat belching, hiccup, and vomiting.

Bladder 47

Located 3 cun lateral to Du 8, at the level of the lower border of the spinous process of the ninth thoracic vertebra.

Functions and Common Usage

Regulates the Liver. Can be used for stomach issues, and difficulty swallowing.

Bladder 48

Located 3 cun lateral to Du 7, at the level of the lower border of the spinous process of the tenth thoracic vertebra.

Functions and Common Usage

Regulates the Gallbladder. Can be used to treat abdominal pain, and jaundice.

Bladder 49

Located 3 cun lateral to Du 6, at the level of the lower border of the spinous process of the eleventh thoracic vertebra.

Functions and Common Usage

Regulates digestion. Can be used to treat belching, and difficult digestion.

Bladder 50

Located 3 cun lateral to the midline, at the level of the lower border of the spinous process of the twelfth thoracic vertebra.

Functions and Common Usage

Regulates digestion.

Bladder 51

Located 3 cun lateral to Du 5, at the level of the lower border of the spinous process of the first lumbar vertebra. Please refer to the image above.

Functions and Common Usage

Regulates digestion.

Bladder 52

Located 3 cun lateral to Du 4, at the level of the lower border of the spinous process of the second lumbar vertebra.

Functions and Common Usage

Strengthens the Kidneys.

Bladder 53

Located 3 cun lateral to the midline, at the level of the second sacral posterior foramen.

Functions and Common Usage
Bladder 53 strengthens the lower back, relieves back pain, and regulates urination. Could be used to treat difficult urination, as well as the inability to urinate.

Bladder 54
Lateral to the hiatus of the sacrum, or the tailbone, 3 cun lateral to Du 2. This point is on the lower back, please refer to the larger Bladder meridian images. The Bladder meridian splits and one line goes down the back of the leg.

Functions and Common Usage
Strengthens the lower back to relieve pain.

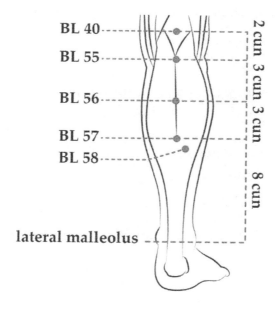

Bladder 55
Located 2 cun below Bladder 40, behind the knee.

Functions and Common Usage
Treats lower back pain.

Bladder 56
Located midway between Bladder 55 and 57, in the center of the belly of the gastrocnemius muscle.

Functions and Common Usage
Bladder 56 treats pain on the Bladder meridian, to relieve back pain. It also treats foot, and heel pain.

Bladder 57
Located directly below the belly of the gastrocnemius muscle, on the line joining Bladder 40 and calcaneal tendon, which is the heel tendon, about 8 cun below Bladder 40.

Functions and Common Usage
Bladder 57 treats lower back pain, heel pain, and calf pain. It also treats hemorrhoids.

Bladder 58
Located 7 cun directly above Bladder 60, on the posterior border of the fibula bone, 1 cun below and lateral to Bladder 57.

Functions and Common Usage
Treats ankle pain, and hemorrhoids.

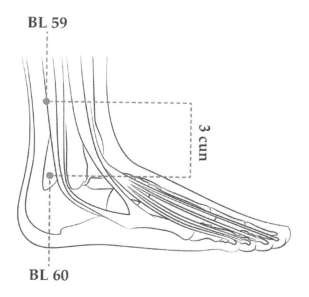

Bladder 59

Located 3 cun directly above Bladder 60.

Functions and Common Usage

Treats lower back pain, ankle pain, and leg pain. Treats back pain that involves the inability to stand back up after sitting.

Bladder 60

In the depression between the lateral malleolus and the calcaneal tendon. Translation: located between the ankle bone on the outside of the ankle, and the tendon on the back of the heel.

Functions and Common Usage

- Ankle pain
- Childhood convulsions
- Headaches on the back of the head, occipital headaches
- Heel pain
- Labor induction, should not be used during pregnancy
- Lower back pain
- Lower leg paralysis
- Neck pain

- Pain in the sole of the foot
- Regulates the Bladder meridian to relieve pain on the meridian
- Relaxes the tendons
- Sacrum pain
- Sciatica
- Seizures
- Severe, sudden back pain that makes walking difficult
- Vertigo

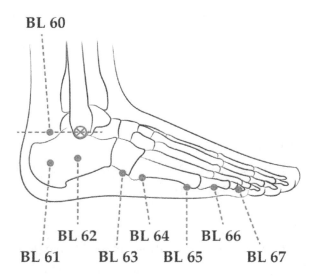

Bladder 61
Located directly below Bladder 60, in the depression of the heel bone at the junction of the red and white skin.

Functions and Common Usage
Treats lower back pain, foot atrophy, heel pain, and foot drop.

Bladder 62
In the depression directly below the lateral malleolus.

Functions and Common Usage
Calms the mind, treats lower back pain, and relaxes the tendons to relieve pain. It treats hemiplegia, stiff neck, epilepsy, and ankle pain.

Bladder 63
Anterior and inferior to Bladder 62, in the depression lateral to the cuboid bone.

Functions and Common Usage
Treats acute back pain. It treats childhood convulsions or seizures.

Bladder 64
Below the tuberosity of the fifth metatarsal bone, at the junction of the red and white skin.

Functions and Common Usage
Calms the mind, treats neck stiffness and pain, and lower back pain.

Bladder 65
Posterior to the head of the fifth metatarsal bone, at the junction of the red and white skin.

Functions and Common Usage
Treats lower back pain, headaches, stiff neck, and blurred vision.

Bladder 66
In the depression anterior to the metatarsophalangeal joint. Translation: Located where the toe bones connect to the bones of the feet.

Functions and Common Usage
Calms the mind, treats neck stiffness, and pain.

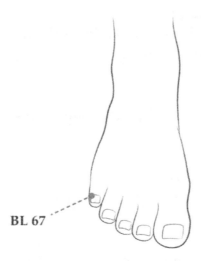

Bladder 67

On the lateral side of the small toe, approximately .1 cun from the corner of the nail.

Functions and Common Usage

Turns the fetus and speeds labor. This point is very famous to turn a breech baby. It is generally treated with moxibustion. Moxibustion is done by burning the herb Mugwort, or Artemisia vulgaris, over the skin. Bladder 67 is listed as treating headaches, and sinus congestion, but it is very popular to turn breech babies.

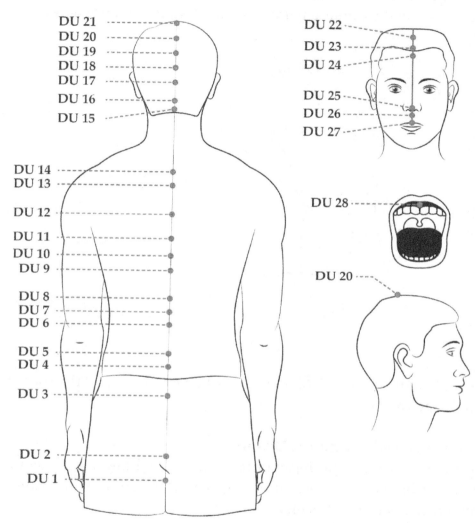

Du Meridian - Governing Vessel

The Du meridian is the Chinese name for the meridian that runs along the spine. It is also called the Governing vessel. It is most commonly referred to by the Chinese name, so that is what I will use here.

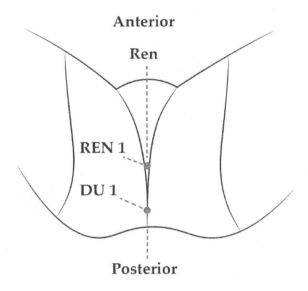

Du 1
Located on the midline (spine) midway between the tip of the coccyx (tail bone), and the anus.

Functions and Common Usage
Treats hemorrhoids, prolapse of the rectum, and lower back pain. This point can be used in cases of emergency when there is an inability to urinate, or retention of urine.

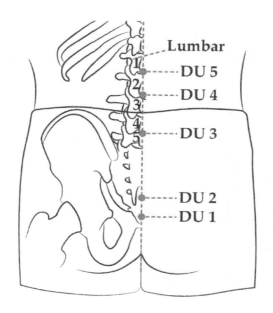

Lumbar
DU 5
DU 4
DU 3
DU 2
DU 1

Du 2
Located at the sacral hiatus, which is a gap on the sacrum (tailbone).

Functions and Common Usage
Treats lower back pain, leg atrophy, and hemorrhoids.

Du 3
Below the spinous process of the fourth lumbar vertebra.

Functions and Common Usage
Strengthens the kidneys, and treats the lower back and legs.

Du 4
Below the spinous process of the second lumbar vertebra.

Functions and Common Usage
Strengthens the kidneys, treats lower back pain, incontinence, and kidney disorders such as nephritis. This is often used to treat lower back pain.

Du 5

Below the spinous process of the first lumbar vertebra.

Functions and Common Usage

Treats lower back pain.

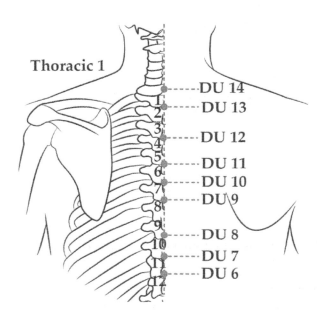

Du 6

Below the spinous process of the eleventh thoracic vertebra.

Functions and Common Usage

Treats lower back pain.

Du 7

Below the spinous process of the tenth thoracic vertebra.

Functions and Common Usage

Treats lower back pain and stiffness.

Du 8
Below the spinous process of the ninth thoracic vertebra.

Functions and Common Usage
Treats back stiffness, and epilepsy.

Du 9
Below the spinous process of the seventh thoracic vertebra.

Functions and Common Usage
Regulates the liver and gallbladder to treat disorders like jaundice, and gallstones. Treats pain and stiffness in the back. Improves circulation in the chest.

Du 10
Below the spinous process of the sixth thoracic vertebra.

Functions and Common Usage
Regulates and opens circulation in the chest to treat cough, and asthma. Treats back and neck pain and stiffness.

Du 11
Below the spinous process of the fifth thoracic vertebra.

Functions and Common Usage
Strengthens the heart, and calms the mind.

Du 12
Below the spinous process of the third thoracic vertebra.

Functions and Common Usage
Regulates the lungs and heart, calms the mind. It opens circulation in the chest and can be used for asthma, bronchitis, coughing, and whooping cough.

Du 13
Below the spinous process of the first thoracic vertebra.

Functions and Common Usage
Strengthens the immune system, regulates the lungs, and clears Heat (Inflammation) from the lungs. Treats cold and flu, and neck stiffness.

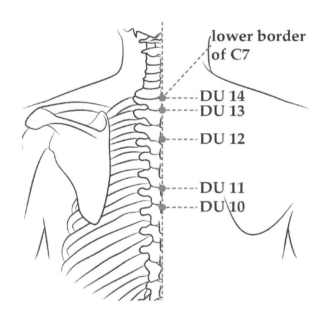

Du 14
Below the spinous process of the seventh cervical vertebra.

Functions and Common Usage
- Back pain
- Calms the mind
- Clears the brain
- Colds and flu
- Spine stiffness in the upper back and neck

This point can treat Lung heat (inflammation). It relieves neck stiffness when you cannot turn your head to the side. It is also listed as treating tuberculosis, emphysema, and hives.

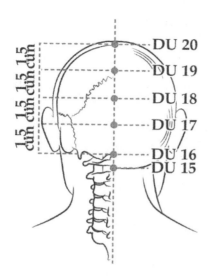

Du 15

One half cun above the posterior hairline, below the spinous process of the first cervical vertebra. It is located opposite the root of the tongue.

Functions and Common Usage

Benefits the tongue. It can be used to treat inability to speak after a stroke, tongue stiffness, and neck pain.

Du 16

Located 1 cun above the posterior hairline, in the depression below the EOP or external occipital protuberance. Translation: On the back of your head there is a little bony area that feels like a knot, that is the EOP.

Functions and Common Usage

Treats neck pain and stiffness.

Du 17

Located 1.5 cun above Du 16, above the EOP or external occipital protuberance.

Functions and Common Usage
This point is called "Brain's Door." It clears the brain and benefits the eyes. It can be used to treat blurred vision, and tinnitus.

Du 18
Located 1.5 cun above Du 17, halfway between Du 16 and Du 20.

Functions and Common Usage
Relieves pain to treat headaches, and calms the mind.

Du 19
Located 1.5 cun above Du 18.

Functions and Common Usage
Relieves pain, and calms the mind.

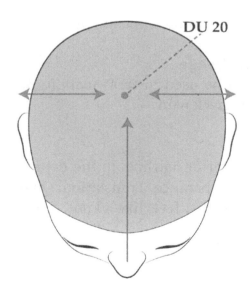

How to Locate Du 20

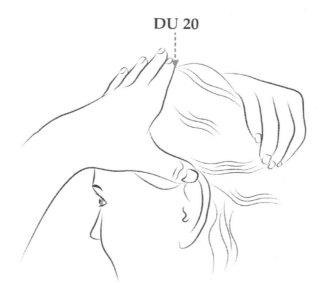

DU 20

Du 20

Located 7 cun above the posterior hairline. You can use your hands to locate this point. Place the tip of your thumbs at the top of your ears, and your fingertips will meet at the top of your head at the approximate location of Du 20. You will feel a slight indentation at the point.

Functions and Common Usage
- Benefits the head and brain
- Calms the mind
- Improves concentration
- Improves memory
- Insomnia
- Opens the sinuses to treat sinus blockage
- Prolapse of the uterus or rectum
- Raises energy and descends it as needed, it regulates circulation
- Restores collapsed Yang
- Revives consciousness

This point can be used to treat prolapse of the rectum, as well as uterine prolapse. It improves memory by increasing blood flow to the brain. It opens the sinuses to treat nasal obstructions that can cause sinus headaches. Collapsed Yang is when the body is so weak that the person faints or passes out.

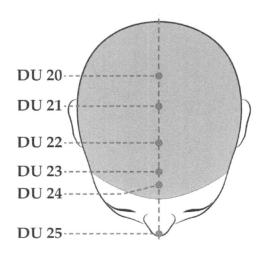

Du 21
Located 1.5 cun in front of Du 20.

Functions and Common Usage
Can be used to treat blurred vision, and nasal discharge.

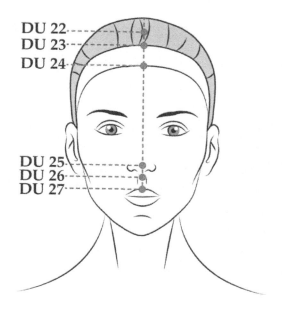

Du 22

Located 3 cun in front of Du 20.

Functions and Common Usage

Benefits the nose to treat sinus congestion and discharge.

Du 23

Located 1 cun above the front hairline.

Functions and Common Usage

Clears the nose to relieve sinus blockage, sinus inflammation, nasal polyps, and the inability to distinguish bad odors. It also treats eye pain, and nearsightedness.

Du 24

Located .5 cun above the anterior hairline.

Functions and Common Usage

Calms the mind, and treats sinus discharge. It stimulates memory according to Giovanni Maciocia.

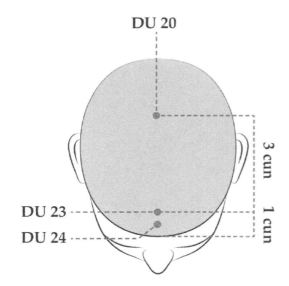

DU 20

3 cun

1 cun

DU 23

DU 24

Du 25
On the tip of the nose.

Functions and Common Usage
Benefits the nose, and restores consciousness.

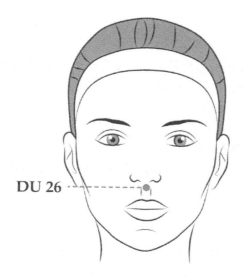

DU 26

Du 26

Above the upper lip, on the midline. Divide the distance between the top of the upper lip, and the border of the nose into thirds. This point is located at the upper third.

Functions and Common Usage

- Acute lower back pain
- Calms the mind
- Clears the nose, treats the inability to distinguish smells
- Coma
- Lockjaw
- Muscle spasms
- Nosebleeds
- Regulates the spine
- Resuscitation point, revives consciousness

Du 26 can be used to treat someone after a stroke or seizure. It strengthens the back to relieve back pain. It can be used to open the sinuses to relieve nasal blockage, and runny nose. This point is the most important point to restore consciousness after fainting or stroke. It can help prevent fainting. If you use acupressure, press strongly, in an upward direction. Using your fingernail, or the tip of your thumb will work best.

Du 27
Located at the top margin of the upper lip. Since Du 27 and Du 28 are not commonly used, I have not included a smaller image of them. You can see the location on the main meridian image.

Functions and Common Usage
This point is not commonly used. It is listed as treating stiff lips, and nosebleeds.

Du 28
Du 28 is located inside the mouth, above the upper teeth, at the border where the upper gums meet the skin of the upper lip.

Functions and Common Usage
This point is not commonly used. It can be used to treat gum disorders.

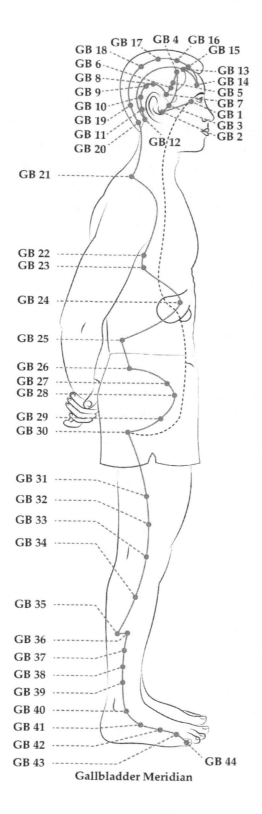

GB 17 GB 4 GB 16
GB 18 GB 15
GB 6 GB 13
GB 8 GB 14
GB 9 GB 5
GB 10 GB 7
GB 19 GB 1
GB 11 GB 3
GB 20 GB 2
GB 12

GB 21

GB 22
GB 23

GB 24

GB 25

GB 26
GB 27
GB 28

GB 29
GB 30

GB 31

GB 32

GB 33

GB 34

GB 35

GB 36
GB 37
GB 38
GB 39
GB 40
GB 41
GB 42
GB 43 GB 44

Gallbladder Meridian

As you can see from the meridian image, this meridian wraps around the side of the head three times. Many of the points on the side of the head are not commonly used. It is hard to describe the location of these points without using anatomy terms. I will highlight, and bullet point the most commonly used points, as usual. Migraine headaches often affect the Gallbladder meridian. It is not common to use the points on the head for migraines. Points on the Liver and Gallbladder meridians on the feet are often used to relieve migraines.

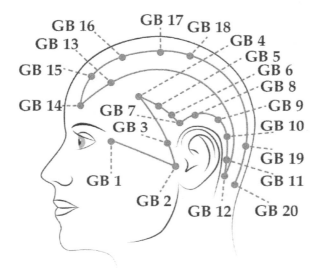

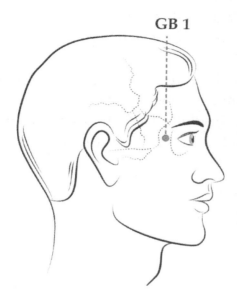

GB 1

Gallbladder 1

Located .5 cun lateral to the outer canthus of the eye, on the bone. In the hollow of the orbital bone.

Functions and Common Usage

- Brightens the eyes
- Cataracts
- Color blindness
- Eye pain
- Farsightedness
- Glaucoma
- Lasik dry eye
- Night blindness
- Optic nerve atrophy
- Retinal hemorrhage

Clinical Notes

This point is very effective to treat dry eyes caused by Lasik eye surgery. It is listed as treating "superficial visual obstruction," which correlates to something affecting the cornea of the eye. When eye surgery is done, the cornea is cut. This severs the nerves in the eye, which means they no longer function normally. This point stimulates normal nerve function in the eyes. This helps to restore healthy eye function.

I find that the eye will usually start watering within a few minutes of treating this point. This is an amazing relief for people with dry eyes due to any cause. If the surgery was done a long time ago, it will usually take longer to see results, and other points would be combined with Gallbladder 1 for better results.

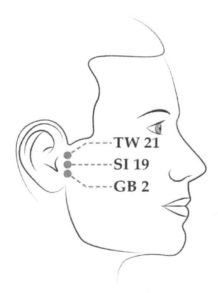

Gallbladder 2
Anterior to the intertragic notch, on the posterior border of the condyloid process of the mandible. Locate with the mouth open. Translation: located in front of the ear. Please see the image for this one.

Functions and Common Usage
Opens the ears to treat deafness, tinnitus, ear infections and discharge, as well as ear pain. Treats hearing loss, jaw pain, and TMJ pain.

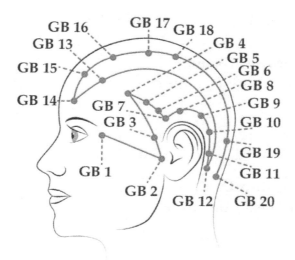

Gallbladder 3

In front of the ear, on the upper border of the cheekbone, in the depression above ST 7.

Functions and Common Usage

Treats ear problems such as deafness, and tinnitus. Treats jaw and tooth pain.

Gallbladder 4

Located inside the hairline, one quarter of the distance between ST 8 and GB 7.

Functions and Common Usage

Treats ear pain, tooth pain, and tinnitus.

Gallbladder 5

Located inside the hairline, halfway between ST 8 and GB 7.

Functions and Common Usage

Treats ear, and tooth pain.

Gallbladder 6
Three quarters of the way between ST 8 and GB 7.

Functions and Common Usage
Treats pain in the outer canthus of the eye.

Gallbladder 7
Inside the hairline, one cun anterior to SJ 20, by the ear.

Functions and Common Usage
Treats swelling of the cheek, and jawbone.

Gallbladder 8
In the small depression, 1 cun above the apex of the ear.

Functions and Common Usage
Treats headaches on the side of the head.

Gallbladder 9
In the depression .5 cun behind GB 8, above the ear.

Functions and Common Usage
Treats headaches.

Gallbladder 10
Behind and above the mastoid process, halfway on the arc between GB 9 and GB 11.

Functions and Common Usage
Treats headaches.

Gallbladder 11
Behind and above the mastoid process, on the line connecting GB 10 and GB 12.

Functions and Common Usage
Treats headaches, tinnitus, deafness, and ear pain.

Gallbladder 12
In the depression behind, and below the mastoid process.

Functions and Common Usage
Calms the mind, treats headaches.

Gallbladder 13
Located .5 cun within the hairline, 3 cun from Du 24.

Functions and Common Usage
Treats headache, vertigo, and epilepsy.

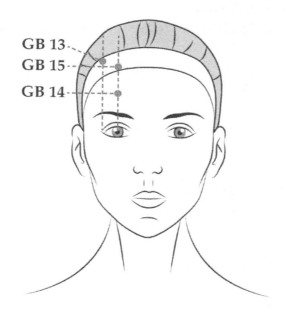

Gallbladder 14
Located on the forehead, 1 cun above the midpoint of the eyebrow.

Functions and Common Usage
- Clears the vision
- Eye pain
- Eyelid drooping
- Eyelid twitching
- Night blindness

Gallbladder 14 treats the eyes, and clears the vision. This is a popular point in cosmetic acupuncture treatments. It lifts the eyelids and improves circulation to the eyes.

Gallbladder 15
Directly above GB 14, .5 cun from the hairline.

Functions and Common Usage
Treats the nose and eyes. Can be used to treat sinus congestion.

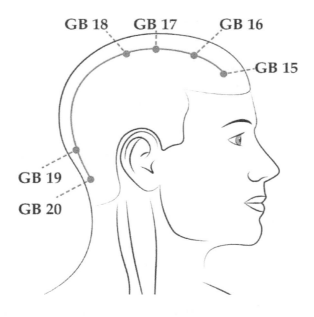

Gallbladder 16
Located 1.5 cun behind GB 15, on the line connecting GB 15 and GB 20.

Functions and Common Usage
Used for all types of eye diseases. Can be used to treat eye pain, and nearsightedness.

Gallbladder 17
Located 1.5 cun behind GB 16.

Functions and Common Usage
Treats headaches.

Gallbladder 18
Located 1.5 cun behind GB 17.

Functions and Common Usage
Treats headaches, and sinus congestion.

Gallbladder 19
Located above GB 20, at the same level as Du 17.

Functions and Common Usage
Treats headaches, neck stiffness, and eye pain.

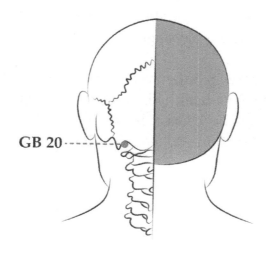

GB 20

Gallbladder 20
In the hollow between the sternocleidomastoid and trapezius muscles.

Functions and Common Usage
- Blurred vision
- Cold and flu
- Dizziness
- Gallbladder meridian pain
- Headaches
- Improves circulation to the eyes
- Loss of speech after a stroke
- Migraines
- Neck pain and stiffness
- Opens blocked ears
- Shoulder pain

Clinical Notes
Gallbladder 20 is very strong to restore normal circulation in the head and neck. It can be used in combination with other points to treat migraine headaches. Most migraines are caused by tight muscles, or blockages in a meridian. The Gallbladder meridian is very commonly affected. Migraines can also be treated by using other points at the opposite end of the Gallbladder meridian, as well as by restoring normal circulation to any area that has a blockage.

Stress causes tight muscles, which then reduce normal blood flow to the brain. Where there is a lack of healthy blood flow, there is pain. It also treats dizziness, which can be caused by tight muscles compressing nerves that affect the ear function.

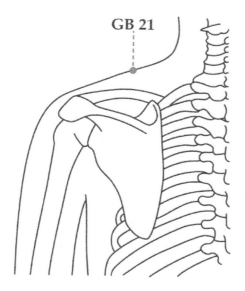

Gallbladder 21

Located halfway between the spine and the tip of the acromion bone.

Functions and Common Usage
- Relieves pain in the neck and shoulders
- Treats breast pain, and breast abscess
- Insufficient lactation
- Should not be used during pregnancy, because it could induce labor

This point is often combined with GB 20 to treat neck pain, because it releases the tight muscles that cause neck and shoulder pain.

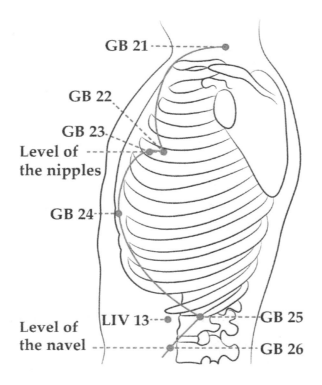

Gallbladder 22

Located 3 cun below the armpit.

Functions and Common Usage

Treats the armpit, and opens the chest. Not used much.

Gallbladder 23

Located 1 cun in front of GB 22, at the level of the nipple.

Functions and Common Usage

Treats chest fullness.

Gallbladder 24

Located below the nipple, in the seventh intercostal space.

Functions and Common Usage
Treats pain in the ribs, mastitis, and hiccups. Regulates the liver, gallbladder and stomach.

Gallbladder 25
On the lower border of the free end of the 12th rib.

Functions and Common Usage
Strengthens the kidneys, treats the lower back.

Gallbladder 26
Below the free end of the 11th rib.

Functions and Common Usage
Regulates menstruation, treats hernia, and abdominal pain.

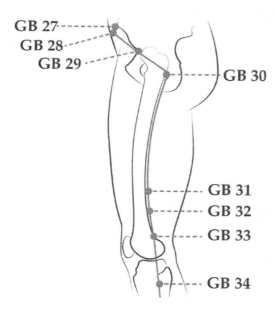

Gallbladder 27
Located 3 cun below the level of the navel.

Functions and Common Usage
Treats uterine prolapse, and abdominal pain.

Gallbladder 28
Located .5 cun in front of and below GB 27.

Functions and Common Usage
Treats uterine prolapse, and abdominal pain.

Gallbladder 29
On the side of the hip joint, at the midpoint between the anterior superior iliac spine, and the prominence of the greater trochanter. Translation: Located on the hip, halfway between the front hip bone and the thigh bone.

Functions and Common Usage
Treats hip pain.

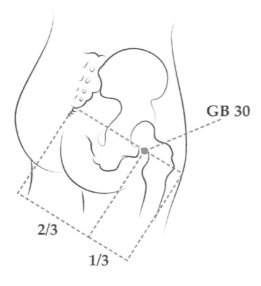

Gallbladder 30

On the back side of the hip joint, one third of the way from the greater trochanter, which is the head of the thigh bone, and the top of the sacrum.

Functions and Common Usage
- Buttock pain
- Hemiplegia
- Hip pain
- Leg atrophy
- Lower back pain
- Sciatica

Clinical Notes

Gallbladder 30 is very effective to treat hip pain, and sciatica. The Gallbladder meridian runs down the side of the leg, to the foot. Sciatica often travels this exact course. It sometimes stops at the knee, but if it is not treated, the sciatic pain can radiate all the way to the foot. Lower back issues must also be considered as a potential factor in hip pain. Herniated discs or tight muscles can easily affect the hip.

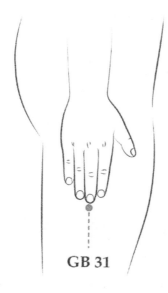

GB 31

Gallbladder 31

On the side of the thigh, 7 cun above the popliteal (knee) crease. Locate where the tip of the middle finger touches the thigh.

Functions and Common Usage

Relieves itching, hives, hemiplegia, knee and thigh pain, and weakness.

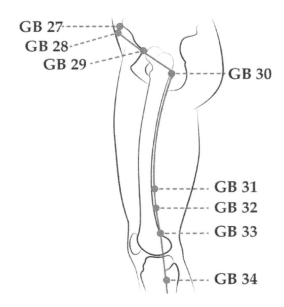

Gallbladder 32

On the side of the thigh, 5 cun above the popliteal (knee) crease.

Functions and Common Usage

Treats pain on the Gallbladder meridian, hemiplegia, hives, and sciatica.

Gallbladder 33
Located 3 cun above GB 34.

Functions and Common Usage
Treats knee pain, relaxes the tendons in the leg, and treats gastrocnemius muscle spasms. The gastrocnemius muscle is on the back of the lower leg.

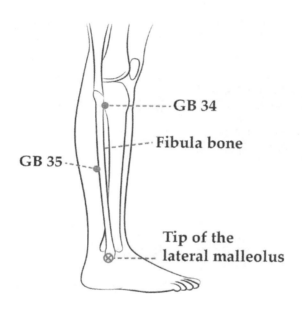

Gallbladder 34
In the depression in front of and below the head of the fibula bone.

Functions and Common Usage
- Calf muscle atrophy
- Contraction of foot tendons
- Hemiplegia
- Hypertension associated with the Liver imbalances
- Knee pain
- Regulates the liver and gallbladder
- Relaxes the tendons to relieve muscle spasms
- Rib pain
- Sciatica

Clinical Notes

This point is used to treat any problem with tendons. It is also used to treat stress, because it treats the Liver, which is associated with stress in Chinese medicine.

Gallbladder 35

Located 7 cun above the tip of the lateral malleolus (ankle bone on the outside of the leg).

Functions and Common Usage

Treats pain on the Gallbladder meridian, relaxes the tendons, treats knee pain, and treats gastrocnemius muscle problems. The gastrocnemius muscles are on the back of the calf.

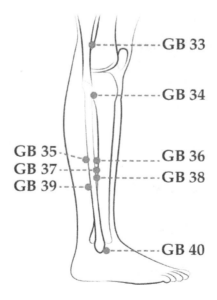

Gallbladder 36

Located 7 cun above the tip of the lateral malleolus, on the anterior border of the fibula bone. (The fibula bone is the small bone behind the tibia bone, which is your calf bone).

Functions and Common Usage
Treats atrophy and pain of the calf, neck pain, and relaxes the tendons.

Gallbladder 37
Located 5 cun above the tip of the lateral malleolus, on the anterior border of the fibula bone.

Functions and Common Usage
- Blurred vision
- Cataracts
- Clears vision
- Eye itching
- Eye pain
- Knee pain
- Lower leg atrophy
- Lower leg pain
- Night blindness
- Optic nerve atrophy
- Regulates the Liver

Gallbladder 37 is the most important point used to treat eye disorders, which is not located directly by the eyes. We call this type of point a "distal" point.

Gallbladder 38
Located 4 cun above and slightly in front of the lateral malleolus, on the anterior border of the fibula bone.

Functions and Common Usage
Regulates the Gallbladder, treats the tendons and bones, and relieves pain on the Gallbladder meridian. It treats the tendons and bones anywhere in the body. It can be used to treat migraines.

Gallbladder 39
Located 3 cun above the tip of the lateral malleolus, behind the fibula bone.

Functions and Common Usage
- Ankle sprain
- Foot weakness
- Leg weakness
- Neck pain and stiffness
- Regulates the Gallbladder

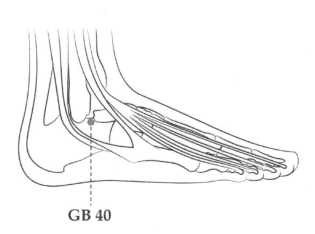

GB 40

Gallbladder 40
Located in front of and below the lateral malleolus (ankle bone on the outside of the leg).

Functions and Common Usage
- Foot drop
- Gallbladder inflammation
- Leg pain
- Lower back pain
- Neck pain
- Regulates the Liver and Gallbladder
- Rib pain
- Wrist pain

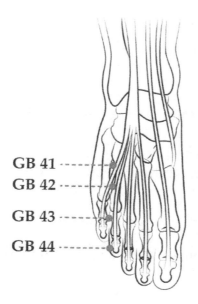

GB 41
GB 42
GB 43
GB 44

Gallbladder 41

Located in the depression between the fourth and fifth metatarsal bones, on the lateral side of the extensor tendon. Translation: Between the fourth and fifth bones of the foot.

Functions and Common Usage
- Foot pain
- Headaches
- Migraine headaches
- Pain on the occiput (base of the skull)
- Regulates the Liver
- Spastic pain of the feet, or toes
- Toe pain

This point can be used to treat many types of headaches, as well as it is listed as facilitating lactation in one source.

Gallbladder 42

Between the fourth and fifth metatarsal bones, on the medial side of the extensor tendon.

Functions and Common Usage

Treats foot pain, rib pain, and headaches.

Gallbladder 43

Between the fourth and fifth toes, at the margin of the toe web.

Functions and Common Usage

Treats headaches, foot pain, vertigo, regulates the Gallbladder, and benefits the ears, and eyes.

Gallbladder 44

On the lateral side of the fourth toe, .1 cun behind the corner of the toenail.

Functions and Common Usage

Regulates the Gallbladder, treats migraines, and vertigo.

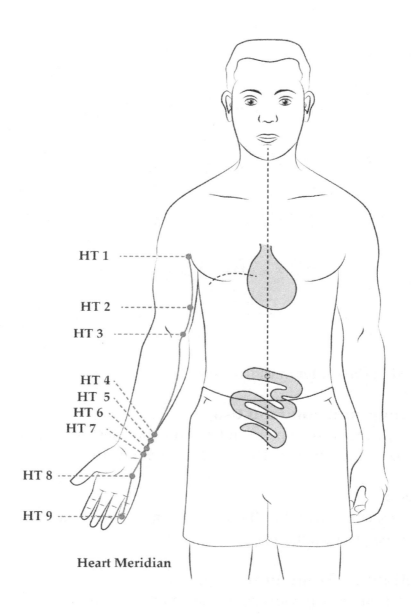

HT 1

HT 2

HT 3

HT 4
HT 5
HT 6
HT 7

HT 8

HT 9

Heart Meridian

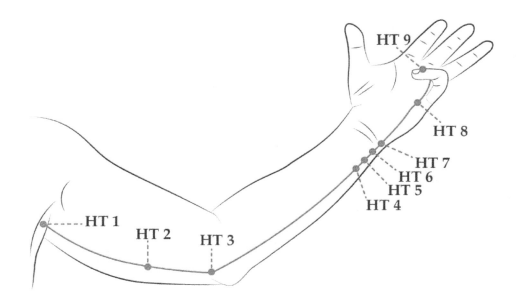

Heart 1
Located in the center of the armpit.

Functions and Common Usage
Regulates the heart, opens and relaxes the chest. Can be used to treat chest pain, and rib pain. This is not commonly used.

Heart 2
Located 3 cun above the elbow crease, in the indentation on the medial side of the biceps muscle.

Functions and Common Usage
Can be used to treat chest pain, and shoulder pain.

Heart 3
Located on the medial end of the elbow crease.

Functions and Common Usage
Heart 3 calms the mind, treats heart pain, and numbness of the hand and arm.

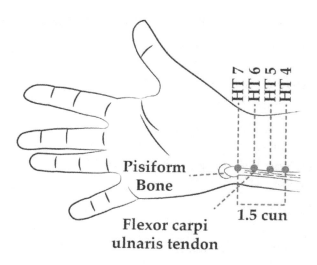

Heart 4

Located 1.5 cun above the wrist crease, on the radial side of the flexor carpi tendon.

Functions and Common Usage

Calms the spirit, treats chest pain, and it can be used to treat sudden loss of voice.

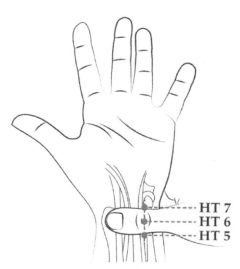

Heart 5
Located 1 cun above the wrist crease, on the radial side of the flexor carpi tendon.

Functions and Common Usage
- Calms the mind
- Heart Fire
- Heart pounding sensation
- Palpitations (when you feel your heart beating)
- Regulates the Heart rhythm
- Strengthens the Heart
- Stuttering
- Sudden loss of voice with tongue stiffness

Heart 5 regulates the heart rhythm, which can treat heart arrhythmia. Acupressure is very effective on this point. Press your fingernail deeply into the point and hold for at least 5 minutes. Regular treatment will regulate and strengthen the heart.

Heart 6
Located .5 cun above the wrist crease, on the radial side of the flexor carpi ulnaris tendon.

Functions and Common Usage
Heart 6 regulates and strengthens the heart, improves circulation to the heart, and cools heat in the blood which could manifest as vomiting blood, or night sweating.

- Heart pain, stabbing pain in the heart
- Night sweating
- Nosebleeds
- Palpitations (when you feel your heart beating)
- Sudden loss of voice
- Vomiting blood

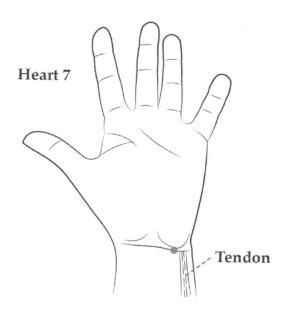

Heart 7

Tendon

Heart 7

Located at the wrist crease, on the radial side of the flexor carpi ulnaris tendon. There might be two wrist creases, and some people have three. This point is located at the level of the largest wrist crease.

Functions and Common Usage

- Anxiety
- Calms the mind
- Heart arrhythmia
- Heart palpitations (you feel your heart beating)
- Heart pounding sensation
- Insomnia
- Irritability
- Manic depression
- Memory
- Regulates and strengthens the Heart

Heart 7 is one of the most important points on the body. It is a top point to treat anxiety and insomnia. It is a very calming point. Acupressure is effective on this point, you can either use your fingernail on this point, or use a magnetic pellet. It treats disorders caused by Heart imbalances, such as poor memory, irritability, and mania.

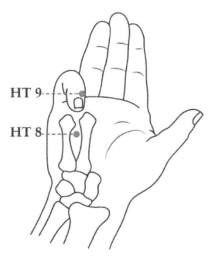

Heart 8

Located between the fourth and fifth metacarpal bones. Locate this point while making a fist. It is located where the little finger touches the palm.

Functions and Common Usage

Heart 8 calms the mind, and regulates the Heart. It can be used to treat palpitations. It treats *Heart Fire*. This is a syndrome that causes extreme irritability, and often insomnia.

Heart 9

Located .1 cun posterior to the corner of the nail on the little finger.

Functions and Common Usage

Revives consciousness, regulates the Heart, and calms the mind. It can be used to treat heart pounding, and heart pain, although Heart 9 is not commonly used.

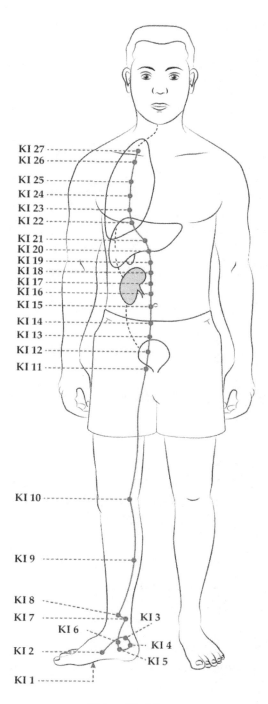

KI 27
KI 26

KI 25
KI 24
KI 23
KI 22

KI 21
KI 20
KI 19
KI 18
KI 17
KI 16
KI 15

KI 14
KI 13

KI 12

KI 11

KI 10

KI 9

KI 8
KI 7
KI 6

KI 3

KI 4
KI 2
KI 5

KI 1

Kidney Meridian

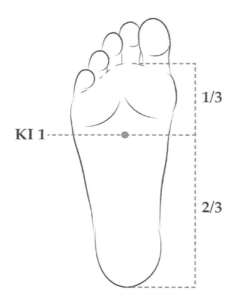

KI 1

1/3

2/3

Kidney 1
Located on the sole of the foot in the depression made when the foot is flexed, at the top 1/3 of the sole.

Functions and Common Usage
Calms the spirit, and revives consciousness. Treats anxiety, insomnia, and headache. This point is used to lower energy that is in excess in the head. It pulls energy down, so it is very relaxing.

Kidney 2
Located in front of and below the medial malleolus, in the depression below the navicular bone tuberosity.

Functions and Common Usage
Strengthens the kidneys, clears heat and fire. Kidney 2 can be used to treat uterine prolapse, and genital itching.

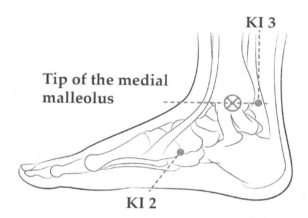

Kidney 3

In the depression between the medial malleolus, which is the ankle bone, and the back of the leg. Locate the point halfway between the tip of the medial malleolus and the back of the leg.

Functions and Common Usage
- Asthma
- Deafness
- Fatigue from Kidney weakness
- Frequent urination
- Heel pain
- Incontinence
- Insomnia
- Memory issues
- Strengthens Kidney Yang, which is associated with urination issues
- Strengthens the lower back and knees, helps to relieve back pain and knee weakness
- Strongly strengthens the kidneys
- Tinnitus
- Urgent urination

- Wheezing

Kidney 3 is the most important point on the Kidney meridian. It is used to treat any type of kidney issue, including frequent or urgent urination, incontinence, waking at night to urinate, and it calms the fetus. It can be used to treat ear disorders like deafness, tinnitus, as well as kidney stones. It can also treat insomnia that is caused by a kidney weakness.

Clinical Notes

In Chinese medicine, the kidneys are the root of health. If you can keep your kidneys strong and healthy, you will live longer and be healthier. The kidneys are also one of the most important things affecting your energy level. Fatigue can be caused by weak kidneys. I like to combine this point with Kidney 7 and Kidney 6 for a stronger effect.

I have used this three point combination, Kidney 3, 6, and 7, to treat a patient who was on kidney dialysis. After a few weeks of treatment, she no longer needed dialysis. These points strengthened her kidneys enough so they could function on their own. I would never make a claim that I can cure kidney disease with these points, but in her case she was able to discontinue her kidney dialysis, after having received that treatment for several years.

Kidney dialysis filters the blood. This is necessary when the kidneys are too weak to sufficiently filter the blood. If you strengthen the Kidneys with acupuncture, the function of the kidneys is improved. Acupressure would be helpful for this. Acupuncture is much stronger, but you can benefit the kidneys by using acupressure on Kidney 3, 6, and 7.

I also used Kidney 3, 6, and 7 on another patient who had kidney problems. She had been told that her kidney function was declining, probably due to a reaction to an antibiotic. Her medical doctor told her she might have to go on dialysis. With weekly acupuncture she had restored kidney health and did not have to go on dialysis.

Something to consider about the kidney points is the effect they have on the emotions. The kidneys are associated with drive and willpower. If your kidneys are weak, you will suffer from fatigue and your drive to get ahead will be reduced. For a severe kidney deficiency, Chinese herbs are very effective to quickly restore the emotional aspect of the kidneys. Weak kidneys can also cause you to feel cold in general, as well as cause hot flashes.

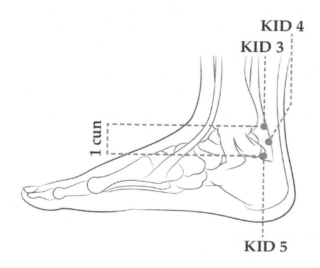

Kidney 4
Located below and behind the medial malleolus, close to the calcaneus tendon.

Functions and Common Usage
- Asthma
- Calms the mind
- Chronic fatigue
- Constipation
- Dementia, it clears the brain
- Dry mouth
- Heel pain
- Hot flashes
- Lower back pain

- Mania, and other emotional imbalances
- Painful urination
- Palpitations
- Strengthens the kidneys
- Swallowing difficulty
- Willpower, strengthens the will

Kidney 4 is very calming, and it also improves emotional issues such as willpower. In Chinese medicine, you must have strong kidneys to have healthy energy levels, as well as the motivation and drive needed to push ahead in life. KI 4 calms the spirit, and clears the brain. It can be used for chronic fatigue, heel pain, coughing blood, difficult breathing, and lower back pain caused by kidney weakness. In Chinese medicine theory, the Kidneys are involved in some breathing problems.

Kidney 5
Located 1 cun below Kidney 3.

Functions and Common Usage
Strengthens the kidneys, regulates the bladder, and regulates menstruation. It can be used for irregular menstruation, painful menstruation, uterine prolapse, painful urination, blurred vision, and frequent urination.

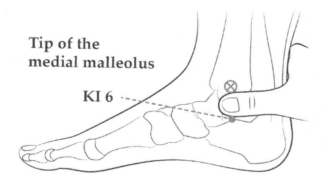

Tip of the
medial malleolus

KI 6

Kidney 6
In the depression of the lower border of the medial malleolus, 1 cun below the medial malleolus, or inner ankle bone.

Functions and Common Usage
- Asthma
- Calms the mind
- Constipation
- Dribbling urination
- Edema
- Expedites labor, do not use during pregnancy
- Frequent urination
- Hot flashes
- Insomnia
- Irregular menstruation
- Moistens the throat
- Sleeping too much
- Sore throat
- Strengthens the kidneys
- Uterine prolapse

Kidney 6 can be used for a sore or dry throat. It is a major point for insomnia, it is very calming. It also treats urinary issues such as frequent urination, and incontinence.

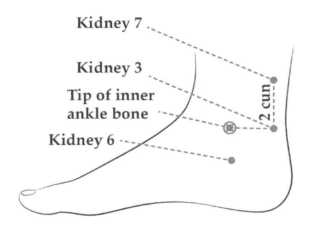

Kidney 7

Located 2 cun above Kidney 3.

Functions and Common Usage

- Dry mouth
- Edema, which is the abnormal retention of fluid causing swelling, often in the ankles and feet
- Foot pain
- Frequent urination due to Kidney weakness
- Incontinence
- Lower back pain
- Nephritis
- Night sweating
- Regulates sweating
- Regulates the bladder
- Regulates urination
- Strengthens the kidneys

Kidney 7 is a major point and it can be used to treat all aspects of the kidneys. It is especially useful to treat incontinence, although Chinese herbs are also very important for this. Edema is caused by your body not being able to get rid of fluid. You can test yourself by pressing firmly on your ankle for 30 seconds. If there is a depression remaining after you remove your finger, this is a sign that you are retaining fluid. It is very important to treat this. It is a sign that something is not functioning properly. Chinese medicine can treat the root cause of this problem.

Kidney 7 is especially used to treat urinary problems, which include painful urination, and nephritis.

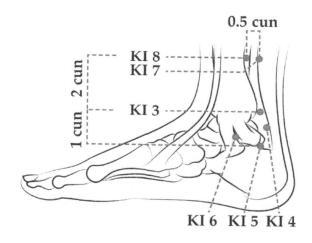

Kidney 8
Located .5 cun in front of Kidney 7, and 2 cun above Kidney 3.

Functions and Common Usage
Kidney 8 strengthens the kidneys, regulates menstruation, stops abnormal uterine bleeding, and also treats uterine prolapse, as well as pain and swelling in the testicles.

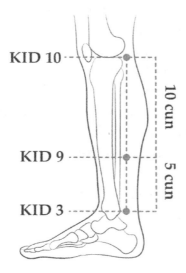

Kidney 9
Located 5 cun directly above Kidney 3, at the lower end of the gastrocnemius muscle.

Functions and Common Usage
Strengthens the kidneys, and calms the spirit. It can be used to treat emotional disorders such as manic depression and mania, although not commonly used for this. It also treats foot pain on the inside arch of the foot.

Kidney 10
Flex the knee to locate, this point is on the inside of the leg, at the end of the knee crease.

Functions and Common Usage
Strengthens the kidneys and clears heat. Can be used to treat genital pain and itching, and knee pain.

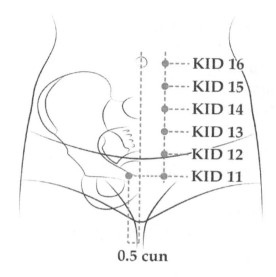

0.5 cun

Kidney 11
Located 5 cun below the navel, on the superior border of the pubic bone, .5 cun lateral to Ren 2.

Functions and Common Usage
This is not commonly used due to the location in the groin area, but could be used to treat uterine prolapse, and urinary disorders.

Kidney 12
Located 4 cun below the navel, .5 cun lateral to Ren 3.

Functions and Common Usage
This is not commonly used due to the location in the groin area, but it could be used for genital issues.

Kidney 13
Located 3 cun below the navel, .5 cun lateral to Ren 4.

Functions and Common Usage
Regulates the lower abdomen. Could be used to treat irregular menstruation, and difficult urination.

Kidney 14
Located 2 cun below the navel, .5 cun lateral to Ren 5.

Functions and Common Usage
Treats the lower abdomen, uterine bleeding, irregular menses, abdominal pain, and distension.

Kidney 15
Located 1 cun below the navel, .5 cun lateral to Ren 7.

Functions and Common Usage
Kidney 15 can be used for irregular menstruation, and abdominal pain.

Kidney 16
Located .5 cun lateral to the navel, at the level of Ren 8, which is at the level of the navel.

Functions and Common Usage
Regulates the intestines to treat constipation and other digestive issues.

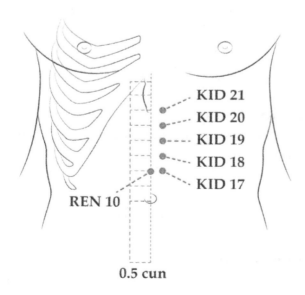

KID 21
KID 20
KID 19
KID 18
KID 17

REN 10

0.5 cun

Kidney 17
Located 2 cun above the navel, .5 cun lateral to the midline.

Functions and Common Usage
This point can be used to treat abdominal pain.

Kidney 18
Located 3 cun above the navel, .5 cun lateral to Ren 11.

Functions and Common Usage
Can be used to treat post-partum abdominal pain.

Kidney 19
Located 4 cun above the navel, .5 cun lateral to the Ren meridian.

Functions and Common Usage
Can be used for abdominal pain or stomach issues such as vomiting or nausea.

Kidney 20
Located 5 cun above the navel, .5 cun lateral to the front midline, or the Ren meridian.

Functions and Common Usage
Regulates the stomach. Can be used for abdominal pain, vomiting, or indigestion.

Kidney 21
Located 6 cun above the navel, and .5 cun lateral to the Ren meridian.

Functions and Common Usage
Regulates the stomach and liver to treat issues such as vomiting, and abdominal pain.

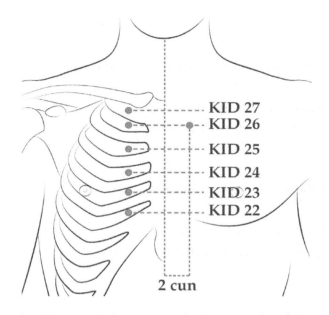

Kidney 22
In the fifth intercostal space, 2 cun lateral to the Ren meridian.

Functions and Common Usage
Improves circulation in the chest. Could be used for cough, or other chest disorders. It is not commonly used due to its location over the lungs.

Kidney 23
In the fourth intercostal space, 2 cun lateral to the midline.

Functions and Common Usage
Regulates circulation in the chest. Could be used for mastitis.

Kidney 25
In the second intercostal space, 2 cun lateral to the Ren.

Functions and Common Usage
Regulates the lungs and stomach. Could be used to treat cough, and chest pain. It is not commonly used due to the location.

Kidney 26
In the first intercostal space, 2 cun lateral to the Ren meridian.

Functions and Common Usage
Regulates circulation in the chest.

Kidney 27
In the depression on the lower border of the clavicle, 2 cun lateral to the Ren meridian.

Functions and Common Usage
Regulates circulation in the chest. Relieves cough and wheezing, although not commonly used. Other points, such as Lung 5, 7, or 9 are more commonly used to treat Lung problems.

The art of healing comes from nature, not from the physician.
Therefore the physician must start from nature, with an open mind.

Paracelsus

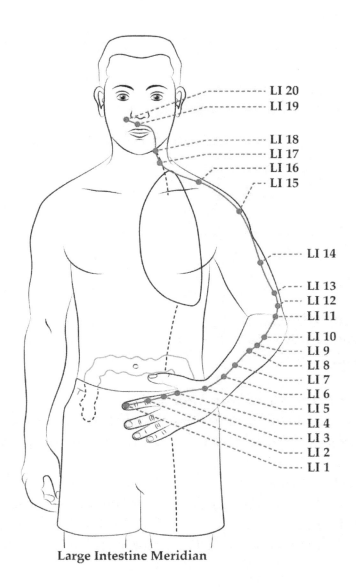

LI 20
LI 19

LI 18
LI 17
LI 16
LI 15

LI 14

LI 13
LI 12
LI 11

LI 10
LI 9
LI 8
LI 7
LI 6
LI 5
LI 4
LI 3
LI 2
LI 1

Large Intestine Meridian

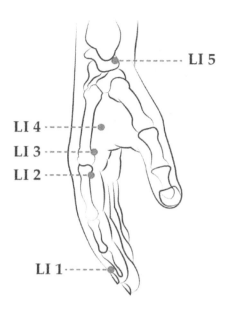

Large Intestine 1

On the radial side of the index finger, about .1 cun posterior to the corner of the nail.

Functions and Common Usage

Revives consciousness, and relieves throat pain by moistening the throat. Can be used to treat toothache, sore throat, and tonsillitis.

Large Intestine 2

On the radial side of the index finger, distal to the metacarpal phalangeal joint, at the junction of the red and white skin. The red and white skin is located just below the bone. The point is located with the finger slightly bent.

Functions and Common Usage

Treats cold and flu, facial paralysis, trigeminal neuralgia, headache, deviation of the eye and mouth, toothache, and sore throat.

Large Intestine 3

On the radial side of the index finger. Make a loose fist, the point is in the depression proximal to the head of the second metacarpal bone.

Functions and Common Usage

Treats cold and flu, trigeminal neuralgia, toothache, tonsillitis, and sore throat. Treats sudden neck stiffness and pain. On source indicates it is very effective for most types of headache. I would combine Large Intestine 3 and 4 to treat headaches with acupressure.

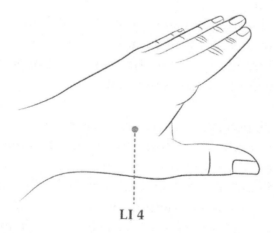

LI 4

Large Intestine 4

Between the first and second metacarpal bones, in the middle of the second metacarpal bone, on the radial side.

Functions and Common Usage
- Allergies
- Arm pain
- Cold and flu
- Constipation
- Deafness
- Ear infections
- Hand pain
- Headaches
- Hives

- Induces labor (it should not be used during pregnancy)
- Nosebleed
- Regulates sweating
- Regulates the face – can treat all face disorders
- Regulates the immune system
- Regulates the Lungs
- Sinus congestion
- Sore throat
- Toothache, lower jaw
- Treats the eyes, nose, mouth, and ears

This is one of the most commonly used points on the body. It is used to treat any issue on the head. It is often combined with Liver 3 to strongly relax the body and balance energy circulation, and relieve pain anywhere in the body. This treatment is called "Four Gates."

Large Intestine 4 is indispensable to treat allergies, and colds and flu. Combine it with Large Intestine 11, Stomach 36, and Stomach 40. Treat every two hours. It boosts the immune system so your body can clear viruses. It treats allergies by regulating and strengthening the immune system, so your body stops overreacting. This is the first choice for acupressure to treat headaches. Acupressure is very effective on this point.

Large Intestine 5
On the thumb side of the wrist. Between the tendons of extensor pollicis longus and brevis. Locate with the thumb tilted upward.

Functions and Common Usage
Treats colds and flu, hives, toothache, sore throat, wrist pain, and calms the mind.

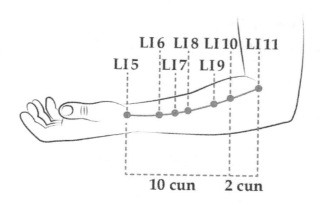

Large Intestine 6
Located 3 cun from LI 5, on the line connecting Large Intestine 5, and Large Intestine 11.

Functions and Common Usage
Clears Heat, or inflammation. Can be used to treat tinnitus, facial paralysis, and tonsillitis.

Large Intestine 7
Located 5 cun above Large Intestine 5, on the line joining LI 5 and LI 11.

Functions and Common Usage
Regulates the Large Intestine. Treats abdominal pain and distention, belching, headaches, and sore throat.

Large Intestine 8
Located 8 cun above LI 5, on the line joining LI 5 and LI 11.

Functions and Common Usage
Regulates the Small Intestine. Can be used to treat abdominal pain, headache, and elbow pain.

Large Intestine 9
Located 3 cun below Large Intestine 11, on the line joining LI 5 and LI 11.

Functions and Common Usage
Regulates the Large Intestine. Can be used to treat shoulder, and elbow pain.

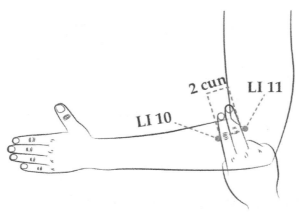

Large Intestine 10
Located 2 cun from Large Intestine 11, on the line connecting LI 5 and LI 11.

Functions and Common Usage
- Arm atrophy
- Arm pain
- Hemiplegia
- Indigestion
- Regulates the intestines
- Regulates the stomach
- Shoulder pain
- Toothache

- Treats arm paralysis after a stroke by strongly stimulating circulation in the Large Intestine meridian

Large Intestine 10 is commonly used to improve circulation in the arm. It can be combined with other points on the meridian such as LI 4, LI 11, and LI 15 to restore healthy blood flow in the arm. Combining points on a meridian is a common way to restore circulation. Using one point alone is often not enough to treat the problem. Strong stimulation of this point can send noticeable warmth to the hands, if they feel cold or the circulation is impaired.

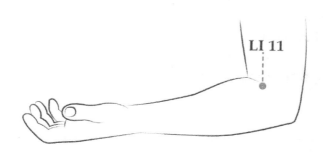

Large Intestine 11
Located halfway between the elbow crease and the elbow. Locate with the arm bent, as shown in the image.

Functions and Common Usage
- Allergies
- Arm atrophy after a stroke, combine with LI 4, LI 10, and LI 15
- Arm numbness
- Arm pain
- Cold and flu
- Constipation – it regulates and moistens the large intestine

- Eczema
- Elbow pain
- Fever reduction
- Heatstroke
- Herpes zoster
- High blood pressure
- Hives
- Itching
- Pain on the Large Intestine meridian
- Psoriasis
- Rashes
- Regulates the Lungs
- Shoulder pain
- Shoulder stiffness
- Skin diseases of all types
- Sore throat
- Strengthens the immune system

Clinical Notes

You can see from the length of this list that Large Intestine 11 is a major point. It clears heat due to many causes, so it treats skin disorders caused by heat, which means inflammatory skin disorders. It is combined with LI 4, ST 36, and ST 40 to resolve colds and flu. It is combined with LI 4 to treat allergies. It is combined with LI 4, SP 6, and LV 3 to treat food allergies. This point combination helps to balance the immune system so it stops overreacting to substances.

Once I had a patient who was very sick, but she refused to see a medical doctor. She was red and very hot, and was showing signs of delirium. I suspected she was dehydrated, and not able to be rational. I used Large Intestine 11 to quickly reduce her fever, and asked her husband to call an ambulance.

This point is very effective when treated with acupressure. I recommend using the thumb to press deeply enough. You will basically be pressing in at the end of the elbow crease.

Large Intestine 11 is the top point to use for constipation. It can be combined with Stomach 36 to regulate the intestines. You can press on both elbows at the same time, or alternate with five minutes on each one. I also use this point to treat patients who have had abdominal surgery. Large Intestine 11 regulates the intestines, which restores normal bowel function after surgery. Surgery disrupts normal intestinal function because the nerves are severed.

Large Intestine 11 is often used in combination with other points on the arm, such as LI 4, LI 10, and LI 15 to restore the function of the arm after a stroke, or after the arm is broken or injured.

This point can be used to treat intestinal problems in babies. It quickly relieves constipation, as well as irregularity of intestinal function. Babies respond quickly to acupressure.

Large Intestine 12
Located 1 cun above Large Intestine 11.

Functions and Common Usage
Can be used to treat arm pain, and elbow pain.

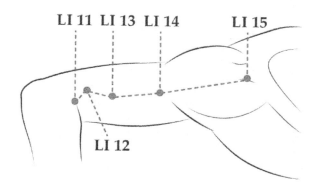

Large Intestine 13
Located 3 cun above Large Intestine 11.

Functions and Common Usage
Can be used for arm and elbow pain.

Large Intestine 14
Located 7 cun above LI 11.

Functions and Common Usage
 Can be used to treat shoulder and arm pain, as well as eye disorders such as conjunctivitis.

Large Intestine 15
Located in front of and below the acromioclavicular joint, which is where your clavicle bone connects with your shoulder, at the origin of the deltoid muscle.

Functions and Common Usage
Commonly used to treat shoulder pain. It can be used in combination with LI 4 and LI 11 to treat arm pain or atrophy. Combining Large Intestine 4, 11, and 15 activates the Large Intestine meridian on the arm, which is very effective to restore normal arm function. This can also be used for stroke recovery.

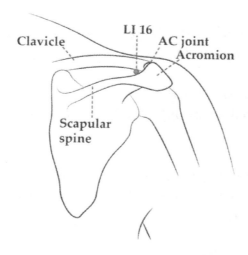

Large Intestine 16

Located on the back side of the shoulder, in the depression between the acromial extremity of the clavicle and the scapular spine. The scapula is commonly called the shoulder blade.

Functions and Common Usage

Can be used for shoulder pain.

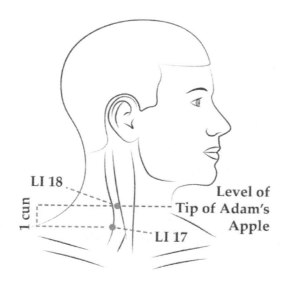

Large Intestine 17

On the lateral side of the neck, 1 cun below LI 18, on the posterior border of the sternocleidomastoid muscle.

Functions and Common Usage

Treats the voice and throat, although rarely used due to the location.

Large Intestine 18

On the lateral side of the neck, at the level of the tip of the Adam's apple, between the sternal head and the clavicular head of the sternocleidomastoid muscle.

Functions and Common Usage

Treats the voice and throat, although rarely used due to the location.

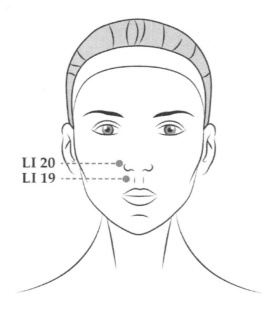

Large Intestine 19

Located below the nostril, .5 cun lateral to the midline.

Functions and Common Usage

Opens the sinuses to treat sinus congestion, and the inability to smell. It is also indicated to treat deviation of the mouth, and Bell's palsy.

Large Intestine 20

Located at the naso-labial groove, at the level of the midpoint of the lateral border of the nostril.

Functions and Common Usage

- Loss of sense of smell
- Mouth deviation, which is when the mouth is crooked due to Bell's palsy or other nerve conditions
- Nasal polyps
- Nosebleeds
- Opens the sinuses
- Sinus headaches
- Trigeminal neuralgia

Large Intestine 20 will open the sinuses to relieve sinus pressure and headaches. It treats loss of sense of smell by opening the sinuses and restoring normal circulation. Mouth deviation and trigeminal neuralgia are treated by the effect this point has on the local nerves. As in all acupuncture, healthy nerve function and circulation are restored, which will treat numerous issues in the affected area.

Natural forces within us are the true healers of disease.

Hippocrates

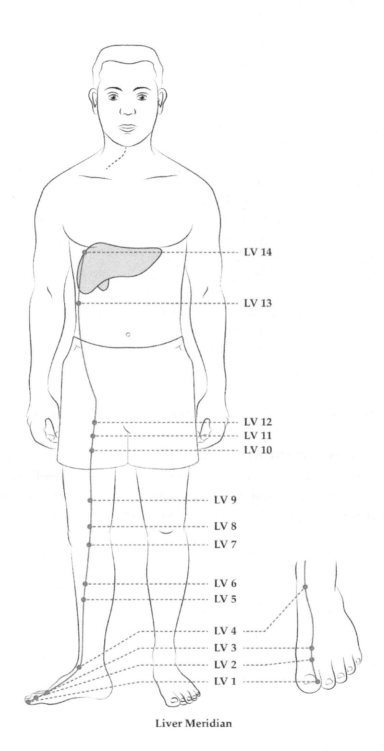

LV 14
LV 13
LV 12
LV 11
LV 10
LV 9
LV 8
LV 7
LV 6
LV 5
LV 4
LV 3
LV 2
LV 1

Liver Meridian

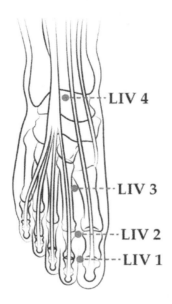

Liver 1

On the lateral side of the big toe, .2 cun from the corner of the toenail.

Functions and Common Usage

Regulates the Liver. Can be used for genital swelling, irregular menstruation, and inguinal hernia. Contains the blood, which means it can be used for all types of abnormal uterine bleeding, as well as blood in the urine or stool.

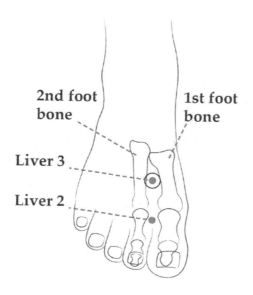

Liver 2
Between the big toe and the second toe, in the web margin.

Functions and Common Usage
- Abnormal uterine bleeding from Fire, which is extreme heat
- Clears Liver Fire
- Convulsions
- Dizziness
- Genital pain
- Headache
- Hepatitis
- Hernia
- Hypertension
- Insomnia
- Jaundice
- Menstrual problems including pain
- Nosebleed
- Regulates Liver Qi
- Seizures
- Severe irritability, with a sensation of heat in the face
- Stops bleeding due to heat syndromes

- Subdues Liver Yang
- Tinnitus
- Treats damp heat in the lower abdomen, this can manifest as many things, including a urinary tract infection
- Treats depression caused by Liver issues

Liver 2 is a major point, it treats symptoms of Liver Fire, and heat in the blood. Bear in mind that some of these symptoms can be caused by other imbalances. Tinnitus, for example, can be related to a Kidney weakness. A full diagnosis must be done for all symptoms.

Liver 2 is a top point for irritability. It strongly purges heat or Fire in the Liver and relieves stress. This point can be combined with Liver 3. It treats the emotions when someone is very irritable, gets a flushed face, or a hot sensation in the face when irritated or stressed. If a person "blows up" or is easily angered, consider using this point. Liver 2 and 3 are used to treat stress, which is caused most often by Liver imbalances in Chinese medicine.

Liver 3

Located between the first and second toes, about 1.5 cun above the web of the toe. Please note that the size of your feet bones determines how far this point is from the toe web, everyone is different. It is located in the depression between the first and second metatarsal bones (bones in the feet).

To locate Liver 3 you can run your finger from the toe web to the foot bones, you will find a small indentation right before you get to the bones of the feet. The image shows the point with a circle around it, so you can see that Liver 3 is located in a small hollow on the foot.

Functions and Common Usage

- Blurred vision
- Dizziness
- Eye conditions
- Frequent sighing

- Headaches
- Hepatitis
- Hernia
- High blood pressure
- Insomnia
- Irregular menstruation
- Jaundice
- Migraine headaches
- Morning sickness
- Nausea
- Regulates blood
- Regulates hormones
- Regulates Liver Qi
- Relaxes the entire body
- Restless fetus disorder, acupuncture helps to calm the baby in utero
- Sedates Liver Yang rising
- Stress relief
- Treats depression caused by stress
- Uterine prolapse
- Vertigo, main point
- Vision problems
- Vomiting

Most people need to have Liver 3 treated. It relieves stress, and it is very relaxing. It treats all diseases that originate in the Liver as viewed by Chinese medicine. It treats migraine headaches and helps to relieve muscle tension. Acupressure is effective on this point. A magnetic pellet can be applied as needed. Remember to remove magnetic pellets after eight hours, or the point will stop responding to treatment temporarily.

Liver Yang rising is often seen in high blood pressure. The stress affects the Liver, which then rises to the head. Controlling anger and high blood pressure are important to prevent strokes. Acupuncture relieves stress, and anger.

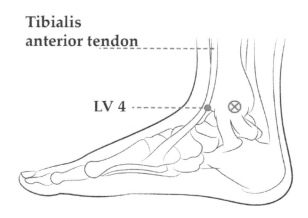

Tibialis anterior tendon

LV 4

Liver 4
Located 1 cun in front of the medial malleolus (ankle bone on the inner ankle). Locate in the depression on the medial side of the tibialis anterior tendon.

Functions and Common Usage
It regulates Liver Qi, and clears heat. It clears heat in the Liver and Gallbladder. It can be used for jaundice, and genital pain.

Liver 5
Located 5 cun above the tip of the medial malleolus, near the medial posterior border of the tibia bone.

Functions and Common Usage
It regulates the Liver, and clears damp heat. It can be used to treat disorders such as hernia, and menstrual issues.

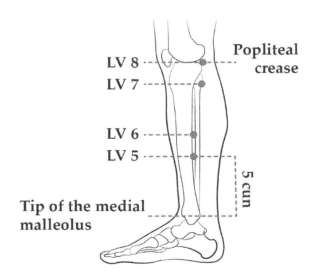

Liver 6
Located 7 cun above the tip of the medial malleolus, near the medial border of the tibia.

Functions and Common Usage
Regulates Liver Qi.

Liver 7
Located behind and below the medial condyle of the tibia, in the upper portion of the medial head of the gastrocnemius muscle.

Functions and Common Usage
Can be used for knee pain.

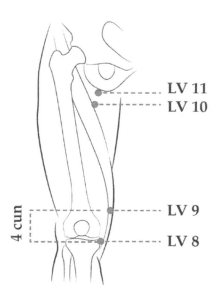

Liver 8

Locate with the knee bent, it is in the depression at the end of the popliteal crease (knee crease).

Functions and Common Usage

Clears damp heat from the lower part of the body, benefits the uterus, and regulates menstruation.

Liver 9

Located 4 cun above the medial epicondyle of the femur.

Functions and Common Usage

Regulates menstruation.

Liver 10

Located 3 cun below ST 30, on the lateral border of the abductor longus muscle.

Functions and Common Usage

Treats abdominal distension, uterine prolapse, and testicle pain.

Liver 11

Located 2 cun below ST 30, on the lateral border of the abductor longus muscle.

Functions and Common Usage
It benefits the uterus, but is not commonly used.

Liver 12

Located inferior and lateral to the pubic symphysis, .5 cun lateral to the Ren meridian, at the inguinal groove. Please refer to the main image for this location. This point is in the pubic area and not commonly used.

Functions and Common Usage
This point could be used for genital issues, but it is not commonly used.

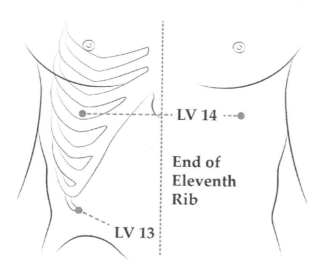

Liver 13

On the lateral side of the abdomen, below the free end of the 11th floating rib.

Functions and Common Usage

It regulates the Liver, and improves digestion.

Liver 14

Directly below the nipple, in the sixth intercostal space.

Functions and Common Usage

It regulates the Liver and Gallbladder. Could be used to treat hepatitis, pancreatitis, and other liver diseases.

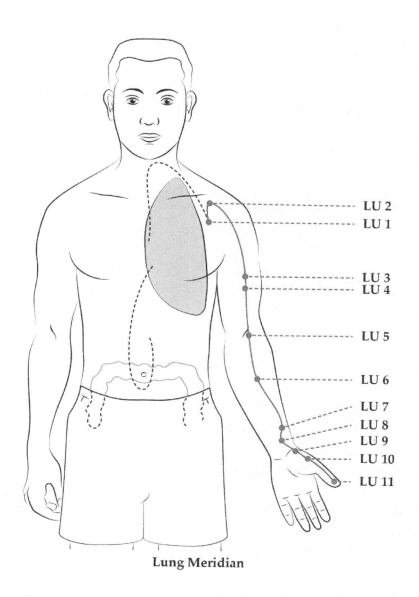

LU 2
LU 1
LU 3
LU 4
LU 5
LU 6
LU 7
LU 8
LU 9
LU 10
LU 11

Lung Meridian

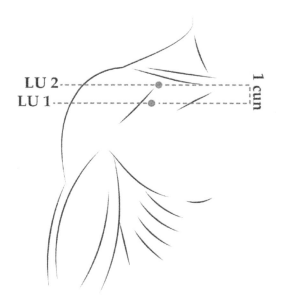

Lung 1

Located latero-superior to the sternum at the lateral side of the first intercostal space, 6 cun lateral to the midline.

Functions and Common Usage

Lung 1 regulates and strengthens the Lungs, relieves cough, wheezing, and difficult breathing. I do not suggest any acupressure be done on the chest or abdomen, unless it is done by a Licensed Acupuncturist. Lung 5, 7, and 9 are more commonly used in the clinic to treat lung issues.

Lung 2

In the depression below the acromial extremity at the clavicle, 6 cun lateral to the midline.

Functions and Common Usage

This point is not commonly needled. It regulates the Lungs.

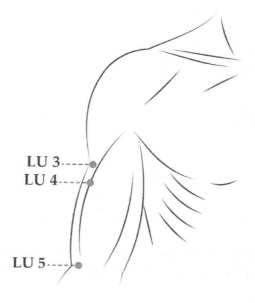

Lung 3

On the medial side of the upper arm, 3 cun below the end of the axillary fold, on the radial side of the bicep muscle.

Functions and Common Usage

Regulates the Lungs.

Lung 4

On the medial side of the upper arm, 1 cun below Lung 3, on the thumb side of the bicep muscle.

Functions and Common Usage

Regulates the Lungs.

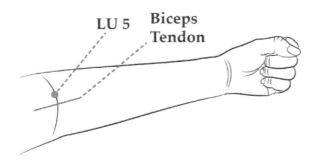

Lung 5

On the elbow crease, on the thumb side of the biceps tendon. Locate the point with the elbow flexed. When you make a fist, the tendon becomes more prominent.

Functions and Common Usage

- Bronchitis
- Clears heat from the Lungs
- Colds and flu
- Cough
- Inflammatory lung conditions
- Regulates the Lung function
- Shortness of breath
- Wheezing

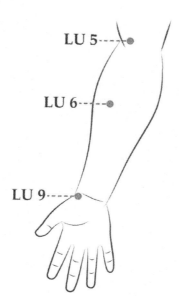

Lung 5 is used to treat inflammation in the lungs. Relieving inflammation will help to relieve the cause of excess mucus production.

Lung 6
On the palm side of the forearm, on the line joining Lung 9 and Lung 5. Located 7 cun above the wrist crease, and 5 cun below the elbow crease.

Functions and Common Usage
Regulates the Lungs, and clears inflammation in the lungs. Could be used to treat asthma, cough, coughing blood, and hiccup.

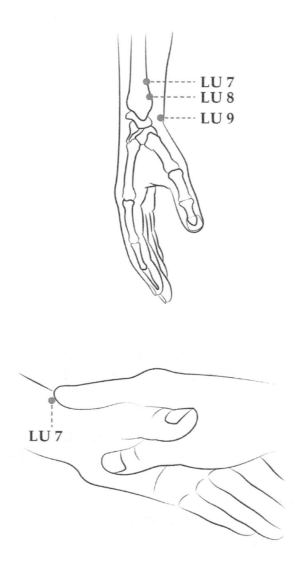

LU 7
LU 8
LU 9

LU 7

Lung 7

Above the styloid process of the radius bone, 1.5 cun above the wrist crease. Located in the depression between the two tendons above the wrist. To locate, place your hands together across each other as shown in the image.

Functions and Common Usage
- Bronchitis
- Mucus or phlegm in the lungs or sinuses
- Regulates and strengthens the Lungs
- Stops coughing – very effective for this, due to any lung problem, including colds and flu, allergies, or asthma
- Wheezing

Lung 7 is a major point that treats coughing, wheezing, and bronchitis with cough. Acupuncture and acupressure can speed up the recovery from colds and flu by stimulating the immune system, and resolving mucus production. It is common to stop coughing within minutes of getting acupuncture on Lung 7. For colds and flu, treat Large Intestine 4 and 11, Stomach 36 and 40. I would recommend treatment at least every two hours. Acupressure is effective on this point.

Lung 8

Located 1 cun above the wrist crease, in the depression on the lateral side of the radial artery.

Functions and Common Usage
Regulates the lungs to treat cough and wheezing.

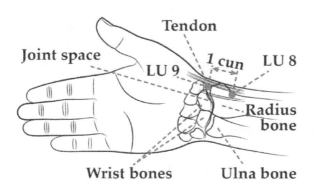

Lung 9

At the thumb side of the wrist crease, in the depression on the lateral side of the radial artery.

Functions and Common Usage

This point strengthens the lungs and resolves mucus in the lungs. It regulates lung function to treat cough, asthma, wheezing, and difficult breathing.

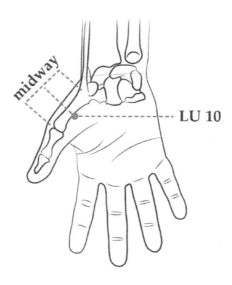

Lung 10

On the radial (thumb) side of the first metacarpal (hand) bone, on the junction of the red and white skin.

Functions and Common Usage

Clears heat in the lungs, which is inflammation. Moistens a dry throat to treat sore throat, hoarseness, and loss of voice.

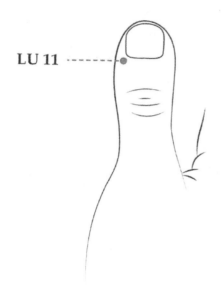

LU 11

Lung 11

On the radial side of the thumb, .1 cun posterior to the corner of the nail.

Functions and Common Usage

Clears Lung Fire (intense inflammation), treats cold and flu, and revives consciousness.

Reality is merely an illusion, albeit a very persistent one.

Albert Einstein

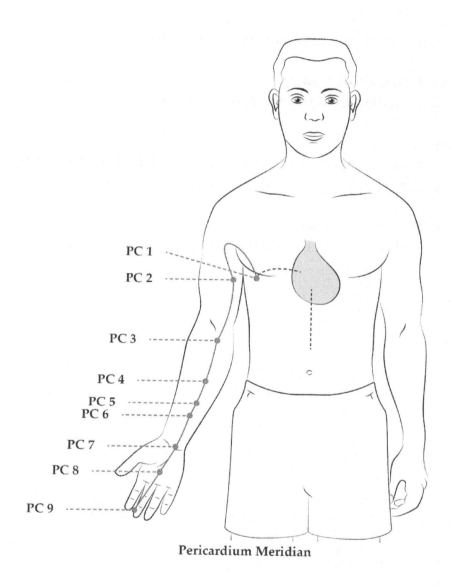

PC 1
PC 2
PC 3
PC 4
PC 5
PC 6
PC 7
PC 8
PC 9

Pericardium Meridian

Pericardium 1

In the fourth intercostal space, 1 cun lateral to the nipple.

Functions and Common Usage

Restores healthy circulation in the chest, benefits the breast.

Pericardium 2

Located 2 cun below the level of the anterior axillary fold, which is the under arm area, between the two heads of the biceps muscles.

Functions and Common Usage

Restores healthy circulation in the chest, relieves pain in the chest.

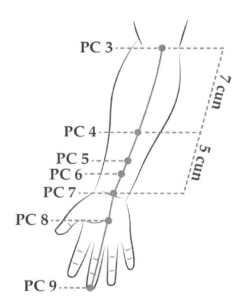

Pericardium 3

On the elbow crease, on the ulnar side of the biceps tendon. (Ulnar side is the little finger side of the arm). Locate with the elbow slightly bent.

Functions and Common Usage

Regulates the Heart, restores circulation in the chest. Cools heat in the blood, which treats hives, and fever.

Pericardium 4

Located 5 cun above the wrist crease, on the line connecting Pericardium 3 and 7, between the tendons.

Functions and Common Usage

Regulates the Heart, calms the spirit, and cools heat in the blood, which can cause coughing of blood.

Pericardium 5

Located 3 cun above the wrist crease, between the tendons.

Functions and Common Usage

Regulates and strengthens the Heart, clears Heart Fire, calms the spirit, transforms phlegm in the heart. This point is indicated in the classics for mania, hysteria, and hallucinations. These mental issues are always treated via the root cause. The imbalance in the Heart causes the mental issues. When the Heart is treated, the emotional issues can be relieved.

Pericardium 5 is also indicated for drooling caused by a stroke. Acupuncture is very effective to help with all aspects of stroke recovery. The patient should get acupuncture as soon as possible after a stroke. Full function can often be restored quickly.

Acupuncture can restore nerve function before the muscles start to go flaccid. Once the muscles have gone flaccid, it will take longer to recover, but there would still be a lot of benefit. If the muscles are not used, they become weak, and recovery requires exercise. Exercise is an important part of recovery after a stroke.

I once treated someone who had a stroke about 18 years prior to getting acupuncture. We were able to warm up his leg, which had remained cold since the stroke. This helped him to walk more comfortably. He was happy to see an improvement. I would suggest that patients who have had a stroke get daily acupuncture as soon as possible after the stroke. I would even suggest twice daily for a week.

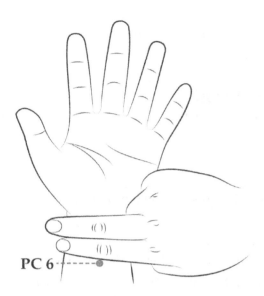

Pericardium 6

Located 2 cun above the wrist crease, between the tendons in the middle of the forearm.

Functions and Common Usage

- Anxiety, calms the mind
- Calms the stomach
- Expedites and regulates lactation, per one source
- Heart Fire, which causes emotional disturbances
- Heart pounding, when you feel your heart beating
- Heart rhythm disorders (consider Heart 5 also)
- Hiccups, it relaxes the diaphragm
- Improves chest circulation to treat difficult breathing
- Inability to speak or loss of memory after a stroke
- Insomnia
- Nausea during pregnancy, including morning sickness
- Palpitations (when you feel your heart beating)
- Regulates the Heart
- Regulates the stomach to treat nausea and vomiting
- Relieves heart pain, angina

- Restores healthy circulation in the chest
- Strengthens the Heart
- Very calming emotionally, often combined with Heart 7 to treat anxiety

This point regulates the stomach, as well as the heart, and the entire chest. It is used to treat anxiety, insomnia, emotional disorders, chest pain, palpitations, and chest fullness.

Clinical Notes

This point is one of the most important points on the body. Acupressure is very effective on this point, there are wrist bands for pregnant women to use for morning sickness that apply gentle pressure to this point all day to relieve nausea. I would recommend alternating wrists for this. The points will not be as responsive if they are continually stimulated. You can put the wrist band on one arm for the day or as needed, then switch to the other arm the next day. Acupuncture is very effective to treat the causes of morning sickness.

Insomnia Point

Acupressure done with a magnetic pellet is very effective to treat insomnia. Just place the magnetic pellet on the point an hour or so before bed, and take it off in the morning. It will help you get to sleep, and stay asleep all night.

Pericardium 6 is famous for treating nausea due to any cause, it regulates the Stomach. It opens the chest to relieve chest pain. Be sure to seek qualified care for any chest pain. Chest pain can be caused by many things, including heart attacks, hiatal hernia, acid reflux, and other digestive issues.

It is sometimes difficult to diagnose the cause of chest pain, because it has so many possible causes. This point relieves chest pain, because it regulates the entire chest. Knowing the cause is not always necessary with acupressure. You can just use the points and allow your body to regulate itself.

If you are taking a boat trip, you can put a magnetic pellet on Pericardium 6 to prevent seasickness.

Please note that this point is located 2 cun above the wrist crease. This is two fingers. If you see an image of three fingers being used to measure it, the last knuckle on the three fingers should be used, not the biggest part of the fingers. There are many images online that are incorrect. It can be tricky to measure. You need to use the patient's fingers to measure. The wrist and hand have to be held at the same level, or the point will be located in a different place.

The easiest way to locate Pericardium 6 is to just use two fingers at the largest knuckles. If you bend your hand back at the wrist, the point location will be slightly off. If you measure the point correctly, mark the spot with a pen, then tilt your hand back, you will see it is in a different location.

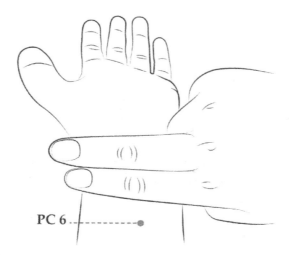

Wrong location!

Notice how the point is too far from the wrist crease. The reason I had this image made is that this is the most common mistake patients make when I show them how to find the point. If you keep your hand at the same level as your arm, and do not bend it back at the wrist, you will locate the point easily.

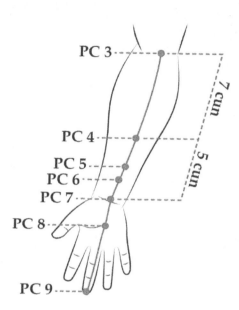

Pericardium 7

In the middle of the wrist crease, between the tendons.

Functions and Common Usage

Regulates the heart, treats insomnia, and regulates the stomach.

Pericardium 8

On the palm, between the second and third metacarpal (hand) bones. Locate with a clenched fist, where the point is below the tip of the middle finger.

Functions and Common Usage

Regulates the heart, clears Heart Fire, revives consciousness, and clears the brain.

Pericardium 9

In the center of the tip of the middle finger.

Functions and Common Usage

Restores consciousness. Some sources say it is effective to restore the ability to speak after a stroke.

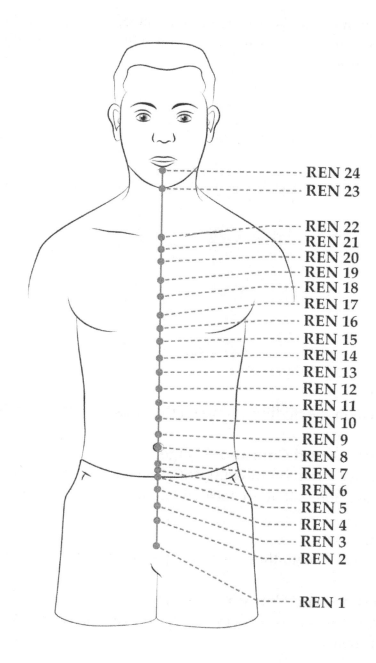

REN 24
REN 23

REN 22
REN 21
REN 20
REN 19
REN 18
REN 17
REN 16
REN 15
REN 14
REN 13
REN 12
REN 11
REN 10
REN 9
REN 8
REN 7
REN 6
REN 5
REN 4
REN 3
REN 2

REN 1

Ren Meridian - Conception Vessel

The Ren meridian is also called the Conception Vessel. The abbreviation for Conception Vessel is CV, so you will see this meridian under both those names.

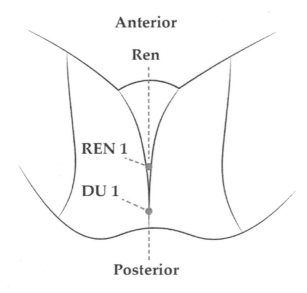

Ren 1
Located on the midline, between the anus and the genitals.

Functions and Common Usage
Can be used to treat difficult urination and incontinence, although there are other points that are located on the arms and legs to treat this.

Ren 2
Located on the midline, on the upper border of the pubic symphysis.

Functions and Common Usage
Treats urinary disorders such as the inability to urinate, and incontinence.

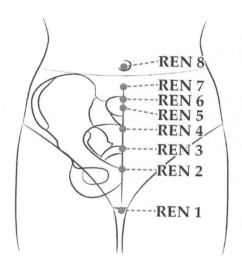

Ren 3
Located 4 cun below the navel, on the midline.

Functions and Common Usage
Treats bladder issues, regulates the uterus, strengthens the kidneys, and treats abdominal pain.

Ren 4
Located 3 cun below the navel, on the midline.

Functions and Common Usage
- Fatigue
- Infertility
- Lower back pain
- Regulates the lower abdomen
- Regulates the small intestines
- Regulates the uterus
- Restores the Yang after collapse, this is a Chinese medicine description of what happens when the energy levels of the body are so low that the person suffers a complete collapse
- Strengthens the kidneys

- Strongly boosts deep energy levels
- Treats the bladder
- Urinary incontinence
- Urinary retention due to fetal pressure

This point is an important point to treat fatigue. It also treats infertility, and regulates menstruation. It restores the body after a collapse of the Yin or Yang, which can manifest as a stroke, coma, or collapse. It raises the energy of the body, so it can be used to treat organ prolapse such as rectal or uterine prolapse, although Chinese herbs would be very helpful to treat this.

Ren 5
Located 2 cun below the navel, on the midline.

Functions and Common Usage
Regulates the uterus, strengthens the kidneys, and treats difficult urination.

Ren 6
Located 1.5 cun below the navel, on the midline.

Functions and Common Usage
- Kidney stones
- Rectal prolapse
- Regulates the Ren meridian
- Regulates urination
- Restores collapsed Yin or Yang
- Strengthens the kidneys
- Tonifies Qi and Yang to treat fatigue
- Uterine prolapse

Ren 6 is a major point. It is used to improve energy levels, as well as treat prolapse of the uterus, rectum, and vagina. A prolapse is when the organ slips down from its normal position. In Chinese medicine theory, organ prolapse is caused by weak energy levels that cause your body to not be able to hold organs in their proper locations. Chinese herbs are often used for this also. There are herbal formulas that not only strongly boost energy, but that lift the energy to treat prolapsed organs. Chinese tonic herbs are very effective to restore energy levels.

Ren 7
Located 1 cun below the navel, on the midline.

Functions and Common Usage
Ren 7 regulates menstruation and can be used to treat abnormal uterine bleeding, vaginal itching, and discharge.

Ren 8
Located in the center of the navel, on the midline. Ren 8 is not treated with acupuncture, instead moxibustion is used. There are many types of moxa. Moxa is the herb mugwort, it can be rolled into a stick and lit on one end to apply stimulation to points. Moxa can also be placed on top of a slice of ginger root to enhance the warming effect of the treatment.

Functions and Common Usage
Ren 8 can be used to restore consciousness, which could be caused by a stroke. It can also be used to treat weak digestion in children. The image below shows a moxa stick being used to warm the lower back. Moxibustion, which is the use of burning moxa, is especially good to treat people after a stroke, because the limbs are often cold. Moxa warms the limb to quickly restore normal blood flow. A lot of acupuncturists are allergic to Moxa smoke. I personally use a far infrared heat lamp. It penetrates the skin and relieves pain.

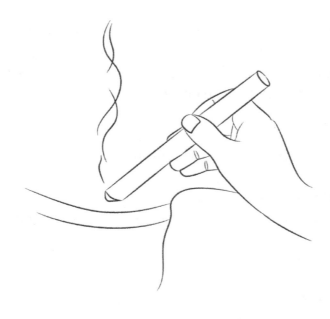

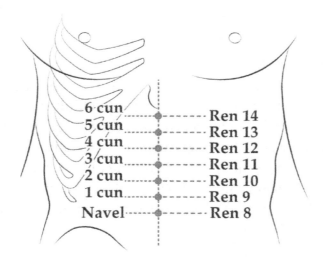

Ren 9
Located 1 cun above the navel, on the midline.

Functions and Common Usage
Regulates the intestines, and can be used to treat abdominal pain.

Ren 10
Located 2 cun above the navel, on the midline.

Functions and Common Usage
Regulates the Spleen and Stomach, which treats digestive disorders such as gastritis, epigastric pain, indigestion, and abdominal pain. It regulates digestion to treat indigestion, and vomiting of food that has not been digested properly.

Ren 11
Located 3 cun above the navel, on the midline.

Functions and Common Usage
Regulates the Spleen and Stomach to treat digestive disorders.

Ren 12
Located 4 cun above the navel, on the midline.

Functions and Common Usage
- Abdominal pain
- Acid reflux
- Burning pain in the throat and esophagus from acid reflux
- Clears Stomach Fire and heat, which is an inflammation of the stomach
- Descends Stomach Qi
- Gastritis
- Hiccups
- Regulates digestion
- Strengthens the Spleen and Stomach to improve digestion
- Treats stagnant digestion
- Ulcers
- Undigested food in the stool
- Vomiting

Ren 12 is a major point to regulate digestion. The stomach is supposed to digest food and send it to the small intestine. If it gets stuck in the stomach and it cannot be digested, it can cause acid reflux, hiatal hernia, and vomiting. Stomach Fire symptoms are similar to gastritis. The stomach feels like it is on fire. Ren 12 clears that type of inflammation.

Ren 13
Located 5 cun above the navel, on the midline.

Functions and Common Usage
- Acid reflux
- Heart pain
- Nausea
- Regulates the Heart
- Regulates the Stomach
- Stomach Fire

Ren 13 can be used to treat gastritis, ulcers, chest pain, and vomiting.

Ren 14
Located 6 cun above the navel, on the midline.

Functions and Common Usage
- Benefits the diaphragm
- Calms the mind
- Opens the chest
- Regulates the Heart
- Regulates the Stomach

Ren 14 regulates the Heart to treat chest pain, but it also treats emotional disorders such as fear, depression, and anxiety. It benefits the diaphragm and can be used to treat disorders such as acid reflux, vomiting, and difficulty swallowing.

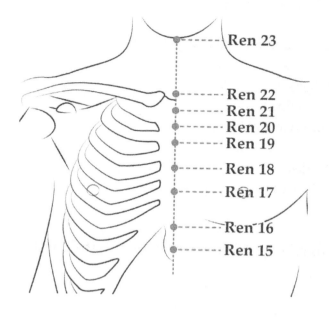

Ren 15
Located 7 cun above the navel, on the midline, below the xyphoid process.

Functions and Common Usage
Regulates the Heart. Regulates circulation in the chest to treat chest distension, acid reflux, pericarditis, and palpitations

Ren 16
Located on the midline of the sternum, at the level of the fifth intercostal space.

Functions and Common Usage
Regulates circulation in the chest.

Ren 17
Located at the level of the fourth intercostal space, on the midline. This point is located at the level of the nipples.

Functions and Common Usage
- Acid reflux
- Breast disorders such as mastitis, and abscess
- Diaphragm spasms
- Difficult breathing
- Difficulty swallowing
- Esophageal constriction
- Hiccups
- Promotes lactation
- Regulates the Lungs
- Wheezing

Ren 17 can be used to restore healthy circulation in the chest.

Ren 18
Located at the third intercostal space, on the midline.

Functions and Common Usage
Regulates circulation in the chest.

Ren 19
Located at the second intercostal space, on the midline.

Functions and Common Usage
Restores circulation in the chest.

Ren 20
Located at the level of the first intercostal space, at the midpoint of the sternal angle.

Functions and Common Usage
Restores circulation in the chest.

Ren 21
Located 1 cun below Ren 22, on the midline.

Functions and Common Usage
Regulates the Stomach, restores circulation in the chest.

Ren 22
In the center of the suprasternal fossa.

Functions and Common Usage
Regulates the Lungs, and moistens the throat.

Ren 23
Above the Adam's apple, in the depression of the upper border of the hyoid bone.

Functions and Common Usage
Benefits the tongue, not used much.

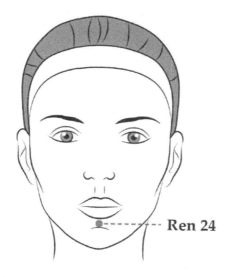

Ren 24

Ren 24
In the depression in the center of the mento-labial groove. Translation: located between the chin and lips, in the middle.

Functions and Common Usage

Relaxes the tendons in the face, can be used to treat deviation of the mouth and eye, lockjaw, facial paralysis, and neck pain.

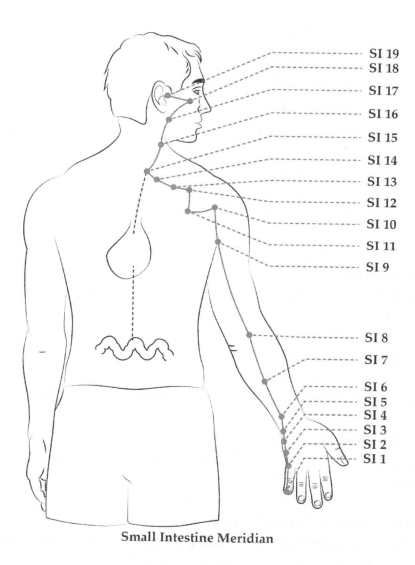

SI 19
SI 18
SI 17
SI 16
SI 15
SI 14
SI 13
SI 12
SI 10
SI 11
SI 9
SI 8
SI 7
SI 6
SI 5
SI 4
SI 3
SI 2
SI 1

Small Intestine Meridian

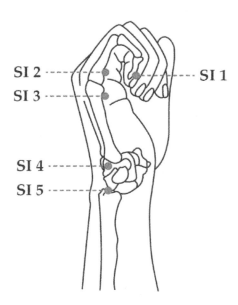

Small Intestine 1
On the ulnar side of the little finger, .1 cun from the corner of the fingernail.

Functions and Common Usage
This point can be used to promote lactation, treat breast abscess, and mastitis. It can also treat loss of consciousness after a stroke.

Small Intestine 2
At the fifth metacarpophalangeal joint (knuckle), locate with the hand in a loose fist.

Functions and Common Usage
This point can be used to treat burning eye pain, and red eyes. Opens the ears to treat deafness, and tinnitus. Moistens the throat.

Small Intestine 3
At the fifth metacarpophalangeal joint (knuckle), locate with the hand in a loose fist.

Functions and Common Usage
- Calms the mind
- Conjunctivitis
- Deafness
- Elbow pain
- Epilepsy
- Eye disorders such as pain, redness, and swelling
- Finger pain
- Hand pain
- Headache on the occiput, or the base of the skull
- Lower back and sacrum pain
- Manic depression, calms the mind
- Neck pain or stiffness
- Regulates the spine
- Relaxes the muscles
- Shoulder pain
- Stiff neck
- Tinnitus
- Upper back pain or stiffness
- Whiplash

Small Intestine 3 is called the "Stiff Neck Point" by many acupuncturists. The indication of manic depression is from the diagnosis of "phlegm heat." This is how Chinese medicine treats emotional disorders. Each emotional imbalance has a root cause, which has a specific diagnosis in Chinese medicine terms. Acupuncture and herbs can be used to treat the underlying imbalance, which can help treat emotional issues that are caused by that imbalance. The diagnosis is made using Chinese medicine diagnosis, not the Western diagnosis.

Small Intestine 4
On the ulnar side of the palm, in the depression between the base of the fifth metacarpal bone, and the triquetral bone.

Functions and Common Usage
Can be used to treat wrist problems including pain, finger and wrist contracture or stiffness. Treats all the fingers, and hand weakness or pain. Relieves neck pain, tinnitus, and jaundice.

Small Intestine 5
On the wrist, in the depression between the head of the ulna bone and the triquetral bone of the wrist.

Functions and Common Usage
Can be used to treat neck pain and swelling, wrist and arm pain. Treats redness of the eyes, deafness, tinnitus, and toothache.

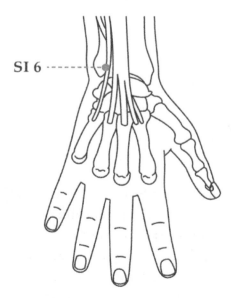

Small Intestine 6
At the head of the ulna bone, on the dorsal side of the wrist.

Functions and Common Usage
Treats pain in the shoulder, upper back, arm, and neck stiffness. Benefits the eyes to treat blurred vision, and eye pain.

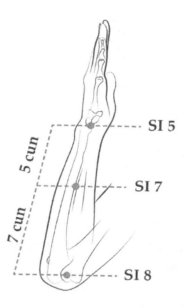

Small Intestine 7
Located 5 cun above SI 5, on the line joining SI 8 and SI 5.

Functions and Common Usage
Can be used to treat finger pain, elbow pain, or pain on the Small Intestine meridian. Treats stiff neck.

Small Intestine 8
Located between the olecranon of the ulna and the medial epicondyle of the humerus bone.

Functions and Common Usage
Can be used to treat elbow and arm pain or stiffness.

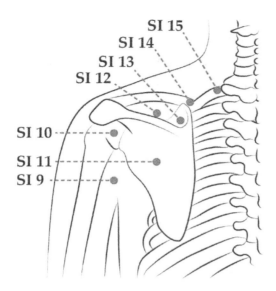

Small Intestine 9
Posterior and inferior to the shoulder joint, located 1 cun above the posterior end of the axillary fold.

Functions and Common Usage
Treats shoulder, and upper arm pain and stiffness.

Small Intestine 10
Directly above SI 9, in the depression inferior to the scapula spine.

Functions and Common Usage
Treats shoulder pain and stiffness.

Small Intestine 11
In the depression on the scapula that is one third from the midpoint of the inferior border of the scapular spine, at the inferior angle of the scapula.

Functions and Common Usage
Treats shoulder pain, insufficient lactation, scapula pain, and restores healthy circulation in the chest.

Small Intestine 12

Directly above SI 11, in the center of the suprascapular fossa, which is the slight indentation on the shoulder blade.

Functions and Common Usage

Treats shoulder and scapula pain, stiff neck, and arm pain.

Small Intestine 13

Located halfway between SI 10 and the second thoracic vertebrae, in the suprascapular fossa.

Functions and Common Usage

Treats shoulder and scapula pain.

Small Intestine 14

Located 3 cun lateral to the lower border of the spinous process of the first thoracic vertebrae.

Functions and Common Usage

Treats shoulder and scapula pain.

Small Intestine 15

Located 2 cun lateral to the lower border of the spinous process of the seventh cervical vertebra.

Functions and Common Usage

Treats shoulder pain. Regulates the lungs, and transforms phlegm to treat asthma, and coughing.

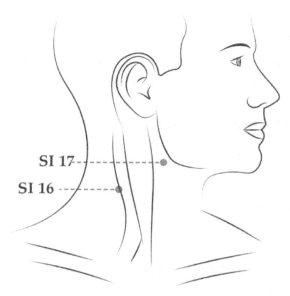

Small Intestine 16

On the side of the neck, on the posterior border of the sternocleidomastoid muscle, at the level of the larynx.

Functions and Common Usage

Treats the ears, and a sudden loss of voice. It is not used much due to the location.

Small Intestine 17

Located between the angle of the mandible, and the anterior border of the sternocleidomastoid muscle.

Functions and Common Usage

Benefits the neck and throat. It can be used to moisten the throat to relieve difficulty swallowing.

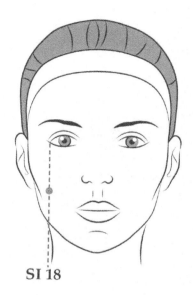

SI 18

Small Intestine 18
Located directly below the outer edge of the eye, in the depression at the lower border of the cheek bone.

Functions and Common Usage
Treats facial paralysis, trigeminal neuralgia, deviated eye and mouth, eyelid twitching, cheek swelling, and toothache of the upper jaw. A deviated eye or mouth are when they are crooked due to muscle tightness, or spasms, which can be caused by a stroke or Bell's palsy.

183

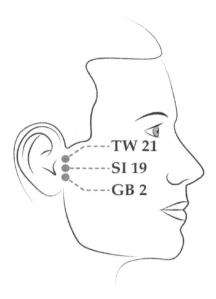

Small Intestine 19

Located in front of the ear tragus, and behind the condyloid process of the jawbone. The depression is more obvious when the mouth is open.

Functions and Common Usage

- Deafness
- Ear discharge
- Ear inflammation
- Headache due to ear issues
- Tinnitus
- Treats the ears
- Vertigo due to ear problems

As you can see in the image, Small Intestine 19 is located in front of the ear, it strongly promotes improved circulation in the ear, so ear disorders can be resolved. Any disorder caused by ear blockage will benefit from improving circulation in the ear.

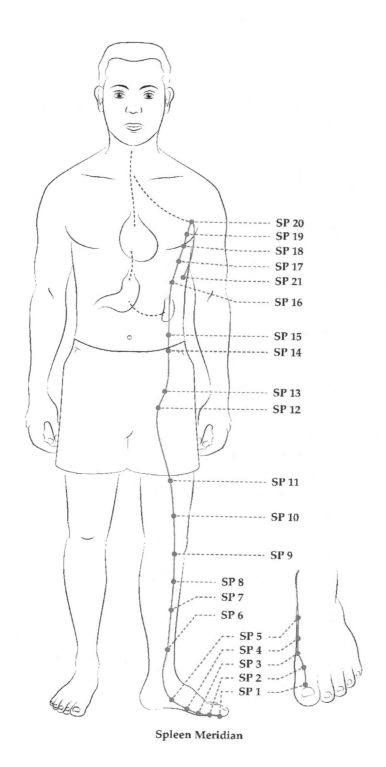

SP 20
SP 19
SP 18
SP 17
SP 21
SP 16
SP 15
SP 14
SP 13
SP 12
SP 11
SP 10
SP 9
SP 8
SP 7
SP 6
SP 5
SP 4
SP 3
SP 2
SP 1

Spleen Meridian

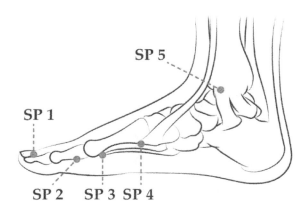

SP 5

SP 1

SP 2   SP 3 SP 4

Spleen 1
Located .1 cun from the corner of the big toenail.

Functions and Common Usage
Stops bleeding, restores consciousness. Can be used to treat uterine bleeding, nosebleed, bloody stools, and vomiting blood. Regulates the Spleen to regulate Blood. It treats bleeding disorders.

Spleen 2
Located on the medial side of the big toe, at the junction of the red and white skin, in the depression between the toe and foot bones.

Functions and Common Usage
Regulates the spleen, resolves digestive disorders such as abdominal distention, belching, and chest oppression caused by digestive problems.

Spleen 3

Located below the head of the first foot bone, by the big toe.

Functions and Common Usage

- Abdominal distension
- Edema
- Fatigue
- Improves digestion
- Nausea
- Strengthens and regulates the Spleen and Stomach
- Toe pain
- Vomiting

Spleen 3 improves digestion and treats edema, which is the retention of excess fluid. It improves energy levels by improving digestion, and the ability to remove excess fluid in the body, which can cause fatigue.

Spleen 4

Located in the depression below the base of the first foot bone, at the junction of the red and white skin.

Functions and Common Usage

Strengthens and regulates the Spleen and Stomach for improved digestion. Regulates digestion to treat indigestion, and vomiting. Regulates menstruation, and treats endometriosis, and morning sickness. Transforms dampness to treat edema, or the retention of excess fluid.

Spleen 5

On the inside of the ankle, below the medial malleolus. Located midway between the tuberosity of the navicular bone, and the tip of the medial malleolus.

Functions and Common Usage
Regulates and strengthens the Spleen and Stomach to treat poor digestion, jaundice, gastritis, and fatigue. Can be used to treat ankle and foot pain. It is also indicated for tongue stiffness.

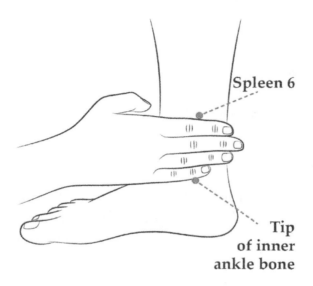

Spleen 6
Located on the inside of the leg, 3 cun above the tip of the medial malleolus, behind the tibia bone. Locate with your whole hand on the tip of the ankle bone. You can easily locate the point by pressing on the area to find the back of the bone.

Functions and Common Usage
- Abdominal distention, bloating in the abdomen
- Amenorrhea – lack of menstruation
- Anemia, blood deficiency in Chinese medicine
- Anxiety
- Balances hormones
- Blurred vision from a Blood deficiency
- Calms the mind
- Dizziness from a Blood deficiency
- Edema, or retention of excess fluid
- Foot paralysis

- Genital pain
- Headache
- Hernia
- High blood pressure that is caused by Kidney deficiency
- Impotence
- Incontinence (combine with Kidney 3, 6, 7)
- Infertility
- Insomnia
- Labor induction, this point should not be used during pregnancy due to its possible effect on inducing labor
- Nourishes the Blood and Yin
- Painful urination
- Promotes urination, causes the body to excrete excess fluid
- Regulates menstruation
- Regulates the blood when it is stagnant, or blood circulation is impaired
- Regulates the Liver
- Relieves pain on the Spleen meridian
- Skin diseases, cools the Blood to treat skin problems like eczema and hives
- Strengthens the Kidneys
- Strengthens the Spleen and Stomach
- Stress
- Urine retention, the inability to urinate
- Uterine prolapse

As you can see from this list of functions and indications, you could almost say that when in doubt, Spleen 6 should be treated. The key things to consider are that it regulates and strengthens the Spleen, Stomach, Kidneys, and the Liver. It treats ailments that have their root in an imbalance in those organs. I would say that it is a rare patient who would not benefit from having this point treated. It is very calming and it treats the underlying cause of insomnia.

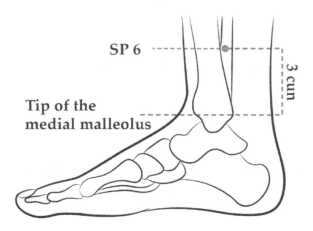

Spleen 6 strengthens the Spleen to encourage the body to get rid of excess fluid. This excess fluid tends to accumulate around the ankles, and on the feet. To test for the presence of edema, press firmly on an area for about a minute. If there is an indentation left behind when you stop pressing that is a sign you are retaining fluid. People often do not notice they have this problem. Acupuncture is very effective to resolve excess fluid. If your finger leaves an indentation, it is called "pitting edema." There is a "pit" where your finger pressed.

Spleen 7
Located 3 cun above Spleen 6, behind the crest of the tibia bone.

Functions and Common Usage
Can be used to treat numbness and pain of the knee and leg, and swelling of the ankles. It tonifies the Spleen to resolve edema.

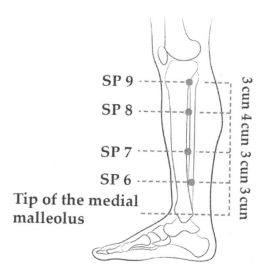

Spleen 8

Located 3 cun below Spleen 9, behind the crest of the tibia bone.

Functions and Common Usage
- Regulates the menstrual cycle
- Strengthens the Spleen
- Regulates the uterus
- Regulates Blood
- Menstrual cramps

This point can be used to treat abnormal uterine bleeding. It is also used to treat painful or irregular menstrual cycles. Menstrual problems can be caused by "stagnant blood" in the uterus. That means that the blood is not flowing properly. This point regulates the blood in the uterus to help resolve menstrual issues.

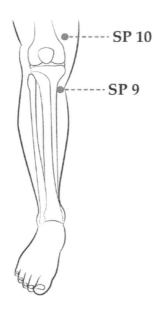

SP 10

SP 9

Spleen 9
Located in the depression by the knee that is at the end of the tibia bone.

Functions and Common Usage
- Abdominal pain
- Edema
- Genital pain
- Knee pain
- Regulates the Stomach
- Strengthens the Spleen

This point is the number one point used to treat edema, or excess fluid anywhere in the body. It encourages the body to expel excess fluid.

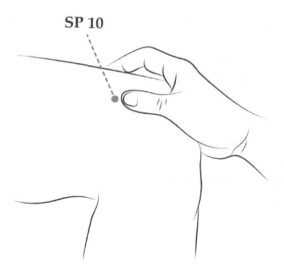

SP 10

Spleen 10

Located 2 cun from the upper border of the kneecap. You can locate this point by cupping your hand over the kneecap. The point is located at the tip of your thumb, on the inside of the leg.

Functions and Common Usage
- Blood disorders
- Cools Heat in the Blood
- Eczema
- Genital itching or pain
- Hives
- Irregular menses
- Itching anywhere on the body
- Knee pain
- Painful menstruation
- Regulates Blood circulation
- Regulates Spleen Qi
- Skin disorders involving heat or inflammation

This point is called the "Sea of Blood." It regulates blood circulation. It is also a cooling point, meaning that it clears disorders that involve inflammation, especially in the skin. It is also used to treat knee pain. It restores healthy blood flow through the knee. The Stomach and Spleen meridians are often used to treat knee pain, because the Spleen meridian is located on the inside of the leg, and the Stomach meridian is on the outside of the leg. Using both of these meridians will encourage healthy blood circulation through the knee.

Spleen 11
Located 6 cun above Spleen 10.

Functions and Common Usage
This point can be used to regulate urination to treat incontinence, or painful urination.

Spleen 12
Located 3.5 cun lateral to the midline, at Ren 2.

Functions and Common Usage
Can be used to treat abdominal pain. This point is located near the genitals and is not commonly used.

Spleen 13
Located .7 cun above SP 12, 4 cun lateral to the midline.

Functions and Common Usage
This could be used to treat abdominal pain, but it is not used much due to its location near the genitals.

Spleen 14
Located 1.3 cun below SP 15, 4 cun lateral to the midline.

Functions and Common Usage
This could be used to treat navel pain, but it is not used much.

Spleen

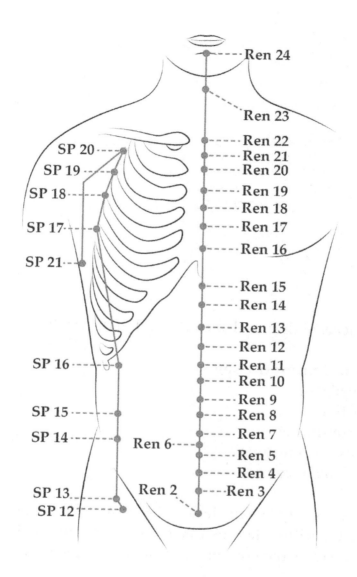

195

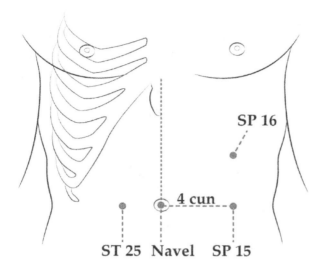

Spleen 15
Located at the level of the navel, 4 cun lateral to the midline.

Functions and Common Usage
- Abdominal pain
- Constipation
- Fecal incontinence
- Regulates the intestines
- Moistens the intestines

This point is used to regulate the intestines. It treats constipation, and it can be combined with other points for constipation such as Large Intestine 11. It restores the normal function of the intestines.

The expression "moistens the intestines" means that it can also treat stubborn constipation, when the stools have dried out. The longer you go without a bowel movement, the drier the stools become. Spleen 15 and Large Intestine 11 are effective to stimulate the Large Intestine, or the colon to empty. Acupressure is effective on both of these points.

Fecal incontinence is when you cannot control your bowels. There are two types of incontinence, urinary and fecal, or stool. Treating your kidneys via Kidney 3, 6, and 7 will treat urinary incontinence. Stomach 36, and Spleen 15 will treat fecal incontinence. These disorders are more common in older age, because the energy of your body naturally declines.

You can avoid incontinence by getting acupuncture to keep everything working properly. I would also suggest Chinese Kidney tonics like Cordyceps. Your acupuncturist will have much stronger Kidney tonic herbs, but Cordyceps can be purchased over the counter to strengthen the kidneys. This will also relieve fatigue.

Spleen 16
Located 3 cun above SP 15, on the abdomen, 6 cun lateral to the midline.

Functions and Common Usage
Regulates the intestines to treat abdominal pain.

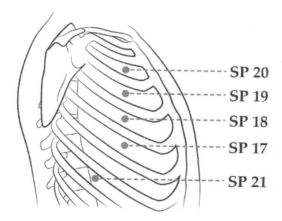

Spleen 17
Located in the fifth intercostal space, 6 cun lateral to the midline. The intercostal spaces are the areas between the rib bones.

Functions and Common Usage
Could be used to improve digestion, but it is not used much.

Spleen 18
In the fourth intercostal space, 6 cun lateral to the midline.

Functions and Common Usage
This point treats insufficient lactation.

Spleen 19
In the third intercostal space, 6 cun lateral to the midline.

Functions and Common Usage
This point could be used to improve chest circulation, but it is not used much.

Spleen 20
In the second intercostal space, 6 cun lateral to the midline.

Functions and Common Usage
This point could be used to treat chest distension, but it is not used much due to the location between the ribs.

Spleen 21
In the seventh intercostal space, in the mid axillary line.

Functions and Common Usage
Regulates circulation in the chest.

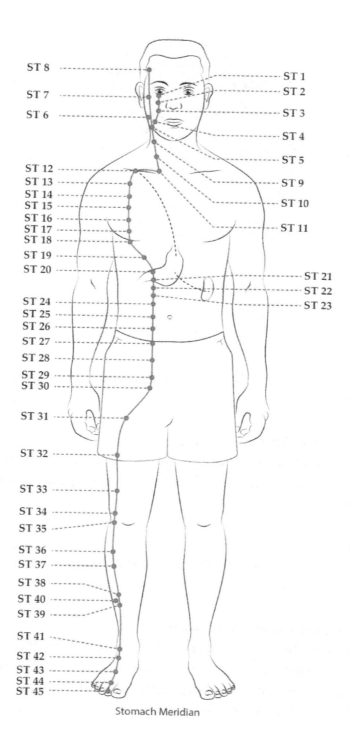

ST 8

ST 7

ST 6

ST 1

ST 2

ST 3

ST 4

ST 5

ST 12
ST 13
ST 14
ST 15
ST 16
ST 17
ST 18
ST 19
ST 20

ST 9

ST 10

ST 11

ST 21
ST 22
ST 23

ST 24
ST 25
ST 26
ST 27
ST 28
ST 29
ST 30

ST 31

ST 32

ST 33

ST 34
ST 35

ST 36
ST 37

ST 38
ST 40
ST 39

ST 41

ST 42
ST 43
ST 44
ST 45

Stomach Meridian

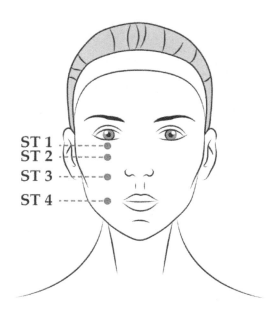

Stomach 1
Located directly below the pupil, inside the orbital ridge, which is the bone for the eye socket.

Functions and Common Usage
Stomach 1 regulates circulation in the eyes, and it can be used to treat all eye disorders including conjunctivitis, eye pain, and excess tear production.

Stomach 2
Located directly below the pupil, on the lower border of the eyeball socket.

Functions and Common Usage
This point can be used instead of Stomach 1 to treat eye diseases. Stomach 2 treats itching eyes, excess tear production, trigeminal neuralgia, conjunctivitis, nearsightedness, eyelid spasm, eye redness and pain, and color blindness. It is listed as expelling parasites, to treat

roundworms in the bile duct. It can open the sinuses to treat sinus headaches, and sinus inflammation.

Stomach 3

Located directly below the pupil, at the level of the lower border of the nostrils.

Functions and Common Usage

Treats facial paralysis, trigeminal neuralgia, eyelid twitching, toothache, swelling of the lips and cheeks, and excess tear production.

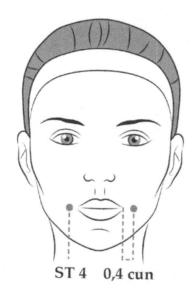

ST 4   0,4 cun

Stomach 4

Located .4 cun lateral to the corner of the mouth.

Functions and Common Usage

Treats facial paralysis, trigeminal neuralgia, excessive saliva production, deviation of the mouth, toothache, eyelid twitching, and inability to close the eye. This point strongly restores circulation in the Stomach meridian to treat disorders of the face. When treating nerve disorders such as facial paralysis, the healthy, unaffected side of the face can also be treated.

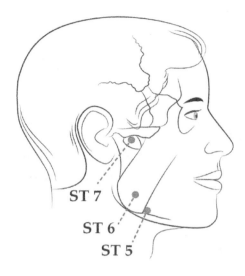

Stomach 5
Located in front of the angle of the jaw, in front of the masseter muscle, in the depression formed when the cheek is bulged.

Functions and Common Usage
Treats facial paralysis, facial pain, lockjaw, facial swelling, mouth deviation, and toothache.

Stomach 6
Located 1 finger width anterior and superior to the lower angle of the mandible, at the prominence of the masseter muscle. Translation: Located in front of and below the angle of the jaw, locate with the jaw clenched, which causes a slight bulge in the muscle.

Functions and Common Usage
Treats facial paralysis, lockjaw, toothache in the lower jaw, sore throat, jaw tension, or TMJ. It clears blockages in the meridian that can be caused by a stroke, or regular jaw clenching. Treats difficulty opening the mouth.

Stomach 7

Located at the lower border of the zygomatic arch, or cheekbone, in the depression in front of the condyloid process of the jawbone.

Functions and Common Usage

- Deafness
- Difficulty opening the mouth, as in lockjaw
- Face pain
- Facial paralysis
- Jaw dislocation
- Tinnitus – ear ringing
- TMJ
- Toothache
- Trigeminal neuralgia

Stomach 7 is located in front of the ear and is very effective to treat jaw disorders. Treating this point will relax the muscles around the jaw and enable the jaw to function normally. Regular teeth grinding or jaw clenching from stress can cause joint problems when tight muscles affect the mobility and alignment of the joint.

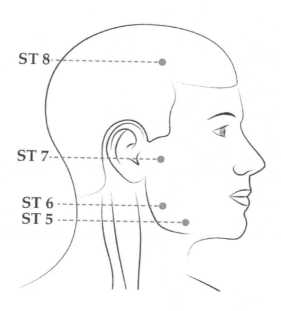

Stomach 8
Located .5 cun from the front hairline, at the corner of the forehead.

Functions and Common Usage
Treats blurred vision, eyelid twitching, and bursting eye pain. It improves circulation in the eyes, and can treat excess tear production.

Note: The points on the Stomach meridian that are located on the neck and chest are not commonly used. I wanted to include them for reference.

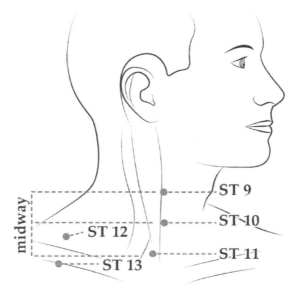

Stomach 9
Located on the neck, 1.5 cun lateral to the larynx.

Functions and Common Usage
Moistens the throat, and can be used to treat difficulty swallowing.

Stomach 10
On the anterior border of the sternocleidomastoid muscle, midway between ST 9 and ST 11.

Functions and Common Usage
Treats sore throat.

Stomach 11
On the medial end of the clavicle, directly below ST 9.

Functions and Common Usage
Treats sore throat.

Stomach 12
Located in the middle of the supraclavicular fossa.

Functions and Common Usage
Treats sore throat, cough, and pain in the supraclavicular fossa, which is the area above your collar bone.

Stomach 13
Directly below Stomach 12, on the lower border of the clavicle bone.

Functions and Common Usage
Treats chest fullness, cough, and asthma.

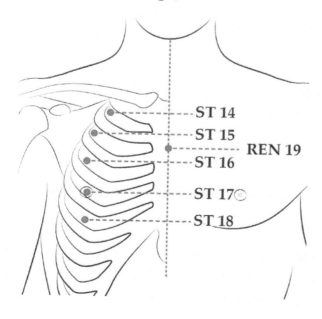

Stomach 14
Located in the first intercostal space, or between the rib bones, 4 cun lateral to the midline.

Functions and Common Usage
Treats chest distension.

Stomach 15
Located in the second intercostal space, 4 cun lateral to the midline.

Functions and Common Usage
Treats breast pain and mastitis. Treats lung disorders such as coughing, wheezing, and shortness of breath.

Stomach 16
Located in the third intercostal space, 4 cun lateral to the midline.

Functions and Common Usage
Treats chest pain, shortness of breath, asthma, and breast disorders such as breast abscess, or mastitis.

Stomach 17
Located at the nipple, in the fourth intercostal space, 4 cun lateral to the midline.

Functions and Common Usage
This point is used as an anatomical landmark, and it is not commonly treated.

Stomach 18
Located in the fifth intercostal space, directly below the nipple.

Functions and Common Usage
Treats insufficient lactation, mastitis, and breast pain. It regulates circulation in the breasts. It improves circulation in the chest to treat coughing, chest fullness, bronchitis, and asthma.

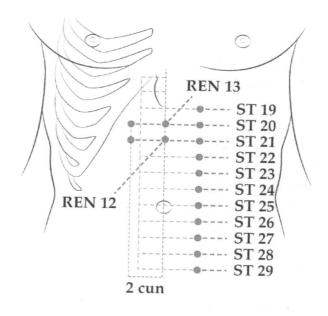

Stomach 19

Located 6 cun above the navel, 2 cun lateral to the midline.

Functions and Common Usage

Treats stomach disorders such as abdominal distension, vomiting, and stomach pain.

Stomach 20

Located 5 cun above the navel, 2 cun lateral to the midline.

Functions and Common Usage

Treats stomach pain, vomiting, and abdominal distension.

Stomach 21

Located 4 cun above the navel, 2 cun lateral to the midline. Located at the level of Ren 12.

Functions and Common Usage

Treats stomach pain, abdominal distension, and vomiting. It regulates digestion.

Stomach 22
Located 3 cun above the navel, 2 cun lateral to the midline.

Functions and Common Usage
Treats abdominal distension, diarrhea, and edema.

Stomach 23
Located 2 cun above the navel, 2 cun lateral to the midline.

Functions and Common Usage
Treats stomach pain, abdominal pain, and diarrhea.

Stomach 24
Located 1 cun above the navel, 2 cun lateral to the midline.

Functions and Common Usage
Treats stomach pain and vomiting. It calms the mind to relieve manic depression. One source indicates it treats manic psychosis. Please remember that Chinese medicine treats emotional disorders via its own system of organ pattern diagnosis.

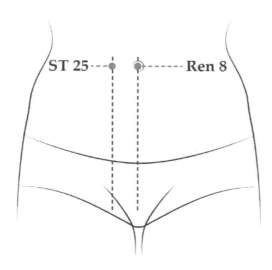

Stomach 25
Located 2 cun lateral to the navel.

Functions and Common Usage
- Abdominal pain
- Appendicitis
- Colitis
- Constipation
- Diarrhea
- Edema
- Intestinal abscess
- Intestinal obstruction
- Moistens and regulates the intestines to treat constipation
- Navel pain
- Pancreatitis
- Regulates digestion
- Regulates menstruation
- Regulates the intestines
- Vomiting

This point should not be used during pregnancy.

This is a major point to treat digestive disorders. It is combined with other points to regulate the intestines, and to treat both constipation and diarrhea. It improves circulation in the intestines, which regulates intestinal function. It can be used after abdominal surgery to restore normal function.

Stomach 26
Located 1 cun below the navel, 2 cun lateral to the midline.

Functions and Common Usage
Treats abdominal pain, hernia, and menstrual pain.

Stomach 27
Located 2 cun below the navel, 2 cun lateral to the midline.

Functions and Common Usage
Treats abdominal distension, and hernia. It strengthens the kidneys to improve urination, and treat painful urination. Treats premature ejaculation, and difficulty urinating.

Stomach 28
Located 3 cun below the navel, 2 cun lateral to the midline.

Functions and Common Usage
Treats retention of urine and stool, painful urination, nephritis, abdominal distension, lower back pain, genital pain, constipation, and painful menstrual cycles. According to one source it expels kidney stones.

Stomach 29
Located 4 cun below the navel, 2 cun lateral to the midline.

Functions and Common Usage
Treats uterine prolapse, vagina pain, infertility, and regulates menstruation. Treats hernia, leukorrhea, and amenorrhea, which is the abnormal absence of a period.

Stomach 30
Located 5 cun below the navel, 2 cun lateral to the midline. Stomach 30 is in the groin area, this point is not commonly used.

Functions and Common Usage
Regulates menstruation, treats infertility, and painful menstrual cycles. One source says it restores the uterus to its normal shape after childbirth. It treats genital pain, and abdominal pain.

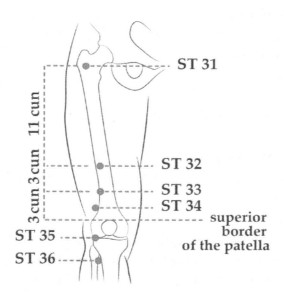

Stomach 31

Located below the anterior, superior iliac spine, at the level of the lower border of the pubis symphysis.

Functions and Common Usage

Treats leg and hip atrophy or paralysis, hip pain, leg pain, numbness and pain in the leg. It can be combined with ST 36, and ST 41 to relieve pain and restore normal leg and hip function.

Stomach 32

Located 6 cun from the kneecap, on the line connecting the anterior, superior iliac spine, and the lateral border of the kneecap.

Functions and Common Usage

Treats knee pain, paralysis of the knee muscles, lower back pain, and hives.

Stomach 33

Located 3 cun from the upper border of the kneecap, on the line between the lateral border of the kneecap and the anterior, superior, iliac spine.

Functions and Common Usage
Relieves lower back pain, weak legs and knees, thigh pain. Treats pain and stiffness of the leg and knee.

Stomach 34
Located 2 cun above the upper border of the kneecap.

Functions and Common Usage
Treats knee pain and swelling, and leg pain. Treats acid reflux, and stomach pain.

This is a major point to treat knee pain. It is often combined with Stomach 35 and 36, as well as Spleen 9 and 10, and He Ding, which is at the top of the knee. Combining these points strongly improves blood flow in the knee to relieve pain and heal the knee after injury, or to treat knee osteoarthritis and prevent the need for surgery. The knee joint is large, and it is easily affected by lack of healthy blood circulation.

One of my patients actually broke his kneecap in half. He had to have surgery to put it back together, but after the surgery, as you can imagine, his knee was very painful. I treated the usual knee points, but he was still in pain. I realized that scar tissue had built up around his kneecap, since it had been immobile for over a month.

The connective tissue on top of the kneecap was either shrunken, or scar tissue was built up, or both. So I did about 30 needles on the top of his kneecap, I just barely inserted the needles into his skin, to penetrate the skin and joint tissue. This is not something you learn in school, you just have to adapt when patients do not respond as expected. After I treated his knee like this, his pain was almost gone.

This case demonstrates why it is important to remember that your acupuncturist will choose the points you need according to her training, and how you respond to each treatment. Each time you get acupuncture, you might have completely different points treated. All types of acupuncture are effective, there are many ways to treat disease with acupuncture.

Stomach 35

Located with the knee bent, this point is at the lower border of the kneecap, in the depression lateral to the patellar ligament. The patella is the kneecap, the patellar ligament is the connective tissue for the kneecap.

Functions and Common Usage

Treats knee pain and swelling, as well as numbness and atrophy of the lower leg.

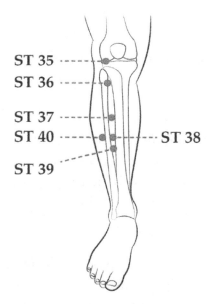

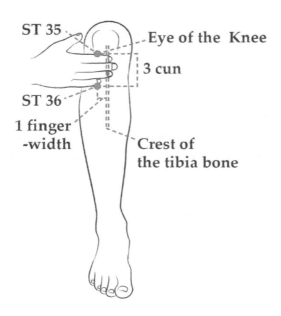

Stomach 36
Located 3 cun below Stomach 35, and one finger width from the anterior crest of the tibia bone.

Stomach 36 can be located several ways. You can place your hand over your knee to measure the point. The index finger is placed at the level of the eyes of the knee, which are the small depressions on both sides of your kneecap. The point is just below your little finger. You can also cross reference the location by using the tibia, or calf bone.

Functions and Common Usage
Stomach 36 is perhaps the most commonly used point in acupuncture. It has so many functions that I will separate the functions from the indications to make it easier to understand. Acupressure is effective on this point.

Regulates and strengthens the Spleen and Stomach
- Abdominal fullness
- Abdominal pain
- Belching

- Constipation
- Diaphragm spasms
- Diarrhea
- Difficulty swallowing
- Edema, fluid retention
- Fatigue
- Gastritis
- Hiccup
- Indigestion
- Mastitis
- Nausea
- Pancreatitis
- Poor appetite
- Prolapse of organs
- Stomach pain
- Vomiting

Regulates and strengthens the Lungs
- Asthma
- Breathing difficulty
- Cough
- Fatigue
- Immune system tonic, can be used for allergies, cold and flu, and general immune system weakness
- Shortness of breath

Regulates and moistens the intestines
- Abdominal pain
- Appendicitis
- Constipation
- Diarrhea
- Enteritis, inflammation of the intestines
- Intestinal abscess

Regulates and strengthens the immune system
- Allergies

- Colds and flu
- Hives

Miscellaneous
- Anemia, helps to build blood
- Benefits lactation
- Blurred vision
- Breast abscess
- Difficulty swallowing
- Dizziness
- Hemiplegia
- High blood pressure, combine with other points to treat the underlying cause
- Knee pain, combined with other points
- Knee weakness
- Leg pain
- Leg paralysis
- Leg weakness
- Leukorrhea
- Mastitis

This point is one of the best points on the body to improve energy levels. It improves digestion, and relieves fatigue. It is called "Leg Three Miles," because the saying goes that even when you are at the point of exhaustion, you can treat this point and walk three more miles.

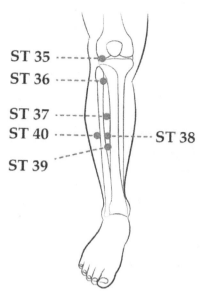

Stomach 37

Located 3 cun below Stomach 36, one finger width lateral to the crest of the tibia bone, which is also called the shin bone.

Functions and Common Usage
- Abdominal pain and distension
- Appendicitis
- Diarrhea
- Enteritis, inflammation of the intestines
- Gastritis
- Indigestion
- Intestinal abscess
- Intestinal obstruction
- Leg pain and numbness
- Leg weakness and atrophy
- Regulates the intestines and stomach
- Resolves stagnation in the intestines

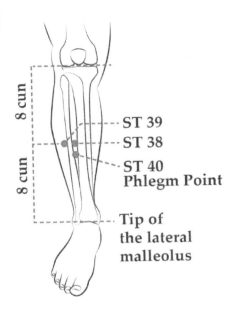

8 cun

8 cun

--- ST 39
--- ST 38
--- ST 40
Phlegm Point

Tip of
the lateral
malleolus

Stomach 38
Located halfway between the eye of the knee, and the tip of the lateral malleolus, which is the ankle bone on the outside of the leg. Located 2 cun below ST 37.

Functions and Common Usage
- Shoulder pain or stiffness
- Lower leg pain or atrophy
- Heat in the soles of the feet
- Foot drop, difficulty lifting the front part of the foot

Stomach 38 treats shoulder pain. In some cases the pain relief is immediate. Additional points can be added to treat the shoulder. Points on the shoulder can be used that restore circulation and help break down scar tissue that often impairs movement.

Stomach 39
Located 3 cun below Stomach 37, one finger width away from the crest of the tibia bone.

Functions and Common Usage
- Regulates the intestines
- Lower back pain referring to the genitals
- Lower abdominal pain
- Breast abscess
- Lower leg pain or paralysis

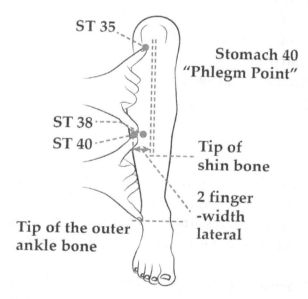

Stomach 40
Located halfway between the eye of the knee and the lateral malleolus, or outer ankle bone. To locate place your little finger over the tip of the outer ankle bone, and the other little finger in the eye of the knee, which is the small indentation by your kneecap. The halfway point is located where your thumbs meet in the middle. The point is located at this level, 2 finger widths from your tibia or shin bone.

Functions and Common Usage
- Asthma
- Bronchitis
- Calms the mind
- Chest or lung problems
- Chest pain from lung issues
- Cold and flu symptoms with excess mucus production

- Cough caused by excess mucus
- Constipation
- Coughing
- Dizziness
- Lower leg pain or paralysis
- Pneumonia
- Regulates the intestines
- Regulates the stomach
- Shortness of breath from mucus in the lungs
- Stomach Fire – gastritis
- Throat pain, obstruction, and swelling
- Transforms phlegm
- Wheezing
- Whooping cough

Stomach 40 is called the *Phlegm Point*. It helps to resolve phlegm, or mucus, anywhere in the body. It is helpful for colds and flu, as it resolves mucus. This point can be combined with Stomach 36, Large Intestine 4 and 11, and Lung 7. This boosts the immune system and resolves phlegm.

People often cancel their acupuncture appointments when they get a cold or flu. Getting acupuncture can help you resolve your cold or flu much faster. I once treated my dad every 2 hours and the next day he was almost symptom free. He had a horrible cough from a cold, and he needed to get well quickly, so I gave him frequent treatments. The next day he rarely coughed and was almost completely well.

When a treatment for excess mucus is given, using Stomach 40, patients often start coughing after the needles are removed. That shows that the mucus in the lungs is being resolved. Your body starts to resolve the mucus by coughing, which is how it expels it. This point can also be used to treat asthma, which is described as the retention of mucus in the lungs, obstructing normal Lung function. It should be combined with other points, and Chinese herbal medicine to treat asthma.

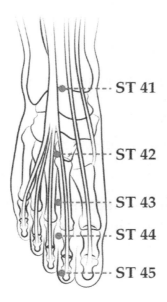

ST 41
ST 42
ST 43
ST 44
ST 45

Stomach 41

Located at the ankle, at the level of the lateral malleolus, or outside ankle bone, in the depression between the tendons.

Functions and Common Usage

- Ankle pain
- Foot drop
- Foot pain
- Headache on the forehead, caused by Stomach issues
- Lower leg pain, atrophy, or stiffness
- Stomach Fire or gastritis

This point is commonly used to restore normal function to the foot, to treat foot pain, or toe pain.

Stomach 42

Located between the second and third foot bones, 1.5 cun from ST 41.

Functions and Common Usage

- Clears heat in the Stomach meridian
- Foot pain or weakness

- Facial paralysis or swelling
- Foot atrophy

Stomach 43
Located between the second and third foot bones.

Functions and Common Usage
- Facial edema, or swelling from excess fluid
- Foot drop
- Foot pain or swelling
- Regulates the spleen to treat edema, or fluid retention
- Regulates the stomach and intestines
- Toe pain or stiffness

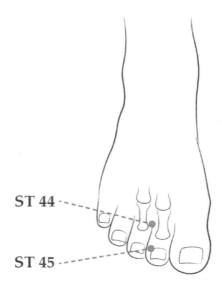

ST 44

ST 45

Stomach 44
Located between the second and third toes, .5 cun from the toe margin.

Functions and Common Usage
- Cold hands and feet when the body is warm
- Constipation
- Diaphragm spasms

- Diarrhea
- Facial paralysis
- Foot pain, or swelling on the top of the foot
- Lockjaw
- Regulates the intestines
- Toothache
- Trigeminal neuralgia

Stomach 45
Located .1 cun from the corner of the second toenail.

Functions and Common Usage
Stomach 45 clears heat from the Stomach meridian, and restores consciousness. Treats facial swelling, and deviation of the mouth, as well as lockjaw.

A person who never made a mistake never tried anything new.

Albert Einstein

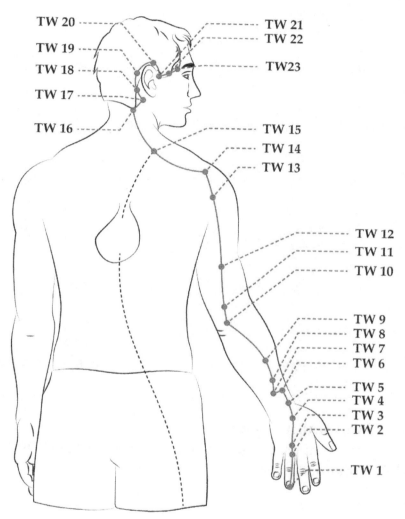

TW 20
TW 19
TW 18
TW 17
TW 16

TW 21
TW 22
TW23

TW 15
TW 14
TW 13

TW 12
TW 11
TW 10

TW 9
TW 8
TW 7
TW 6

TW 5
TW 4
TW 3
TW 2

TW 1

Triple Warmer Meridian

The Triple Warmer meridian is also called the San Jiao meridian. The concept of a Triple Warmer is the ancient way of looking at energy production in the body. There are three warmers, the upper, middle, and lower burners.

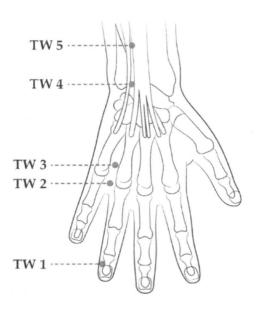

Triple Warmer 1
Located on the top of the ring finger, at the corner of the nail, .1 cun from the corner.

Functions and Common Usage
Benefits the ears and tongue, treats pain on the Triple Warmer meridian. Can be used for tinnitus, deafness, earache, and pain at the root of the tongue.

Triple Warmer 2
Between the ring and little fingers, .5 cun from the web margin on the hand.

Functions and Common Usage
Benefits the ears, treats pain on the Triple Warmer meridian. Treats deafness, earache, headache, dry eyes, and throat pain.

Triple Warmer 3

On the top of the hand, in the depression between the fourth and fifth hand bones.

Functions and Common Usage

Treats the ears, head, and eyes. Treats pain on the Triple Warmer meridian. Can be used for tinnitus (ear ringing), ear blockages, and ear pain. It is considered to be one of the most important distal points to treat ear disorders, due to any cause.

Triple Warmer 4

At the wrist joint, in the depression located lateral to the extensor digitorum communis tendon.

Functions and Common Usage

Relaxes the tendons. Treats arm, shoulder and wrist pain.

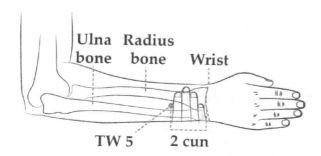

Triple Warmer 5

Located 2 cun above SJ 4, between the radius and ulna bones.

Functions and Common Usage
- Allergies
- Benefits the head and ears
- Colds and flu
- Ear pain
- Headaches
- Hearing impairment

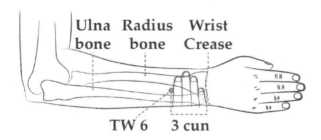

Triple Warmer 6
Located 3 cun from the wrist crease, in the depression between the radius and ulna bone.

Functions and Common Usage
- Benefits the voice
- Constipation
- Opens the intestines
- Sudden loss of voice
- Throat pain
- Tinnitus

Triple Warmer 6 resolves stagnation and opens the intestines. Triple Warmer 6 is used for severe constipation, in combination with other points like Large Intestine 11, and Stomach 36. The points chosen depend on the underlying cause of the problem.

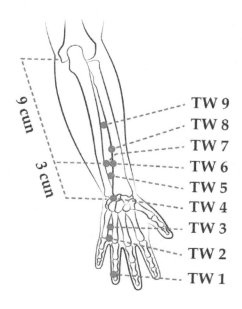

Triple Warmer 7
Located 3 cun from the wrist crease, on the ulnar side at the level of Triple Warmer 4.

Functions and Common Usage
Benefits the ears. Treats deafness, tinnitus, and arm pain.

Triple Warmer 8
Located 4 cun from the wrist crease.

Functions and Common Usage
Clears the meridians and sensory orifices to treat sudden deafness, loss of voice. Treats hand and arm pain.

Triple Warmer 9

Located 7 cun from the wrist crease, in the depression between the radius and ulna.

Functions and Common Usage

Benefits the throat and ears. Used for sudden loss of voice, sudden deafness, tinnitus, and toothache.

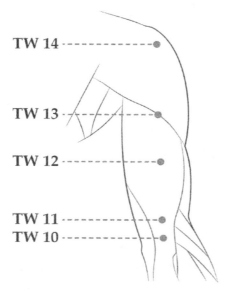

Triple Warmer 10

Located 1 cun from the elbow.

Functions and Common Usage

Activates the meridian and relieves pain. Treats atrophy and numbness of the arm.

Triple Warmer 11

Located 1 cun from Triple Warmer 10.

Functions and Common Usage

Treats pain of the elbow and arm.

Triple Warmer 12
Located halfway between Triple Warmer 10 and 14.

Functions and Common Usage
Treats inability to turn the head, shoulder and arm pain.

Triple Warmer 13
On the posterior border of the deltoid muscle, located two thirds of the distance between Triple Warmer 10 and 14.

Functions and Common Usage
Treats pain of the shoulder and arm.

Triple Warmer 14
Located on the shoulder, 1 cun below LI 15.

Functions and Common Usage
Treats shoulder and arm pain.

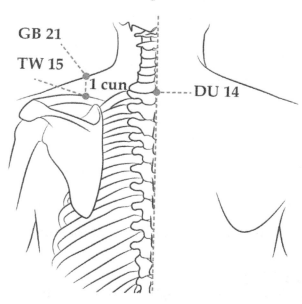

231

Triple Warmer 15
In the suprascapular fossa, in the depression halfway between GB 21 and SI 13.

Functions and Common Usage
Treats shoulder and elbow pain.

Triple Warmer 16
On the posterior border of the sternocleidomastoid muscle.

Functions and Common Usage
Benefits the head and neck. For sudden deafness, headache, and blurred vision. (This point is located on the neck and is not commonly used).

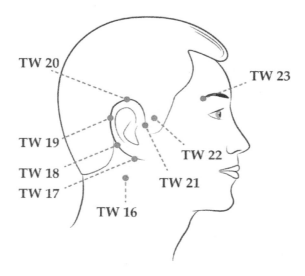

Triple Warmer 17
Located behind the earlobe, between the mandible and mastoid process.

Functions and Common Usage
Benefits the ears, clears heat, and relieves pain on the meridian. Treats deafness, itching inside the ear, redness, pain and swelling of the ear, earache, and tinnitus. Treats lockjaw, and dimness of vision.

Triple Warmer 18
Located in the center of the mastoid process, at the junction of the middle and lower 1/3 of the curve formed by Triple Warmer 17 and 20.

Functions and Common Usage
Benefits the ears. Used for tinnitus, deafness, and ear pain.

Triple Warmer 19
Located behind the ear, at the junction of the upper and middle 1/3 of the curve formed by Triple Warmer 17 and 20.

Functions and Common Usage
Treats the ears. Used for deafness, tinnitus, and ear pain.

Triple Warmer 20
Located directly above the ear apex, which is found by folding the ear forward.

Functions and Common Usage
Benefits the ears and teeth. Treats tinnitus, deafness, toothache.

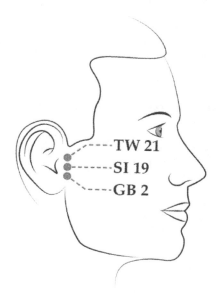

Triple Warmer 21

In the depression in front of the supratragic notch and slightly superior to the condyloid process of the mandible. I know this sounds confusing, but Triple Warmer 21 is at the root of the ear, as shown in the image.

Functions and Common Usage

Treats the ears. Used for tinnitus, deafness, earache. It opens and regulates the ears. It restores normal circulation in the ears, which heals ear disorders.

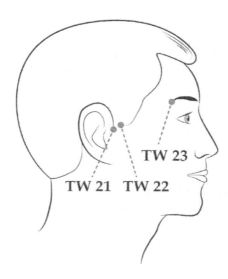

Triple Warmer 22

Located .5 cun in front of the upper border of the root of the ear.

Functions and Common Usage

Treats ear pain, and tinnitus.

Triple Warmer 23

In the depression at the lateral end of the eyebrow.

Functions and Common Usage

Benefits the eyes. Treats blurred vision, eye redness, eye pain, and facial paralysis.

An Mian	Peaceful Sleep
Ba Feng	Eight Winds
Ba Xie	Eight Pathogens
Bi Tong	Penetrating the Nose, or Nose Passage
Dan Nang Xue	Gallbladder Point
Ding Chuan	Calm Difficult Breathing
Er Bai	Two Whites
He Ding	Crane's Summit
Hua Tuo Jia Ji	Hua Tuo's Paravertebral Points
Jia Bi	Sinus Point
Jia Cheng Jiang	Adjacent to Container of Fluids
Jian Qian	Front of the Shoulder
Lan Wei Xue	Appendix Point
Luo Zhen	Stiff Neck
Shi Xuan	Ten Diffusions
Si Shen Cong	Four Alert Spirit
Tai Yang	Supreme Yang
Ti Tuo	Lift and Support
Xi Yan	Eyes of the Knee
Yao Tong Xue	Lumbar Pain Point
Yao Yan	Lumbar Eyes
Yin Tang	Hall of Impression
Yu Yao	Fish Waist
Zi Gong	Uterus Point, also called the Palace of the Child

These points are listed in Chinese first, because they do not have numbers that are commonly used. In most cases the English translation is placed first on the image, but most acupuncturists refer to the points by the Chinese name. These points are called "extra points" because they are in most cases not located on a meridian.

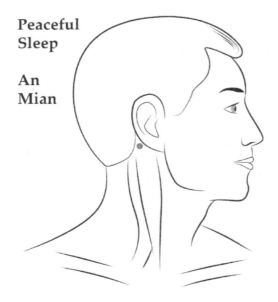

Peaceful
Sleep

An
Mian

An Mian – Peaceful Sleep
At the midpoint between GB 20 and TW 17.

Functions and Common Usage
Calms the spirit. It is used to treat insomnia.

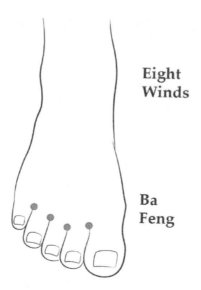

Eight
Winds

Ba
Feng

Ba Feng – Eight Winds

On the top of the foot, between the toes, on the web margins. There are eight points in total.

Functions and Common Usage

Treat foot pain, and headaches. The Ba Feng points are excellent to treat diabetic neuropathy. They work by restoring normal circulation in the feet.

Clinical Notes

Ba Feng are effective to restore healthy circulation in the feet. I use them for diabetic neuropathy or any type of nerve problem in the feet. They are very effective for foot numbness. Patients do not mind them at first, until the nerves wake up and start working again, then they can be sensitive and painful. Once they start to hurt, you know the nerves are working better and you don't need the points as much.

I would also consider using Ba Feng to treat leg problems after a stroke. Treating the ends of the feet is very effective to restore normal nerve function. Acupuncture is preferred, but any type of acupressure will help.

Using a massager in this area, or just massaging the points with your fingers helps.

Eight Pathogens

Ba Xie

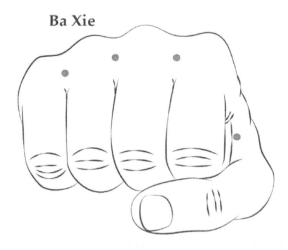

Ba Xie – Eight Pathogens
On the top of the hand, at the junction of the white and red skin of the hand webs. Eight points in all.

Functions and Common Usage
These points treat numbness, stiffness, and pain in the fingers and hand.

Clinical Notes
They are very effective to improve blood flow to the hand and treat and type of hand problem. They also can be used to treat nerve problems. By stimulating the nerves, they regulate nerve function. (When nerves are damaged they tend to misfire. Shooting pains and the loss of control of the hands can be caused by damaged nerves. When the hands are numb, there is a lack of circulation. Stimulating these points encourages restored function). These points correspond to Ba Feng, located between the toes. They both are helpful for nerve diseases.

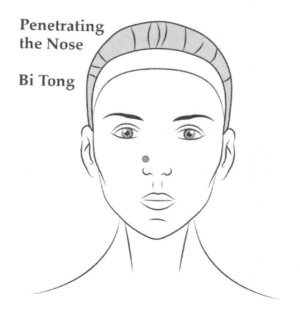

Penetrating
the Nose

Bi Tong

Bi Tong – Nose Passage, or Penetrating the Nose
At the highest point of the nasolabial groove.

Functions and Common Usage
Benefits the nose. Used for sinus congestion and discharge, nasal polyps, allergic reactions. This point stimulates healthy circulation in the sinuses, which is helpful for sinus headaches.

Dan Nang Xue – Gallbladder Point
The tender spot 1-2 cun below GB 34, on the right leg only. Find the most tender spot. GB 34 is located 1 cun below and in front of the head of the fibula bone, by the knee.

Functions and Common Usage
Clears damp heat in the Gallbladder, which treats gallstones, bile duct disorders, and rib pain. Damp heat can be translated as inflammation.

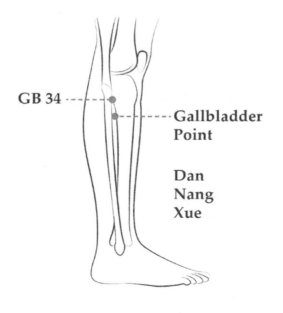

GB 34 - - - - -

- - - - - Gallbladder
Point

Dan
Nang
Xue

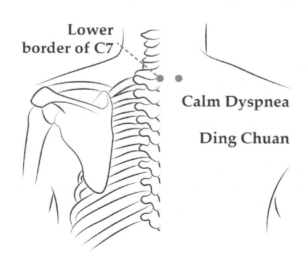

Lower
border of C7

Calm Dyspnea

Ding Chuan

Ding Chuan – Calm Difficult Breathing
Located .5 cun lateral to Du 14, or the level of cervical vertebrae 7.

Functions and Common Usage
Calms difficult breathing, treats wheezing, asthma, and stops coughing.

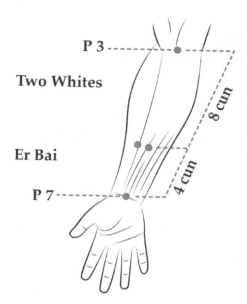

Er Bai – Two Whites

Located on both sides of the flexor carpi radialis tendon, 4 cun from the wrist crease.

Treats hemorrhoids and prolapse of the rectum.

Crane's Summit

He Ding

He Ding – Crane's Summit
In the depression of the midpoint of the superior patellar border.

Functions and Common Usage
Improves blood flow in the knee. This point is combined with other points, like ST 36, ST 35, SP 9 and SP 10 to treat knee pain.

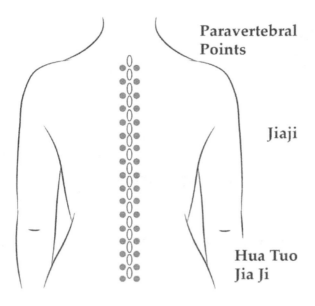

Hua Tuo Jia Ji – Paravertebral Points
A group of 34 points on both sides of the spine, located .5 cun lateral to the lower border of each spinous process. The points run from the first thoracic vertebrae, to the fifth lumbar vertebrae. These points are commonly called the Jiaji points.

Functions and Common Usage
These points can be used to regulate the spinal nerves. They are most commonly used to treat back pain. They strongly stimulate nerve function in the spine to relieve pain, and restore healthy function.

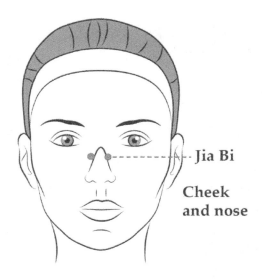

Jia Bi

Cheek
and nose

Jia Bi – Cheek and Nose

Jia Bi is located on the sinus bone, above Bi Tong.

Functions and Common Usage

This point is very effective to open the sinuses. This point is an example of how rich Chinese medicine is. There are so many points that you can learn new ones all the time. I was looking online for an image for Bi Tong, and I found an image that had Bi Tong on it, but it also had a point called Jia Bi. I have never seen this point in a point location book.

I pressed on this point and found it opened my sinuses in seconds. The easiest thing to do is just hold both sides of your nose right at the edge of your sinus bone. You will look like you are holding your nose, but your fingers are higher.

Acupressure is very effective on this point. In fact, I would prefer acupressure over acupuncture on this point. You can press gently on the nose cartilage in this area. This can be used for any sinus blockage. Sinus problems often cause pain anywhere on your face, including sinus headaches. If you have face or jaw pain, consider using these points to restore circulation in your sinuses.

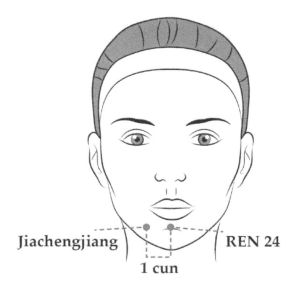

Jiachengjiang   REN 24

1 cun

Jia Cheng Jian – Adjacent to Container of Fluids
Located 1 cun lateral to Ren 24.

Functions and Common Usage
This point can be used to treat deviation of the mouth and eye. It also treats facial paralysis and trigeminal neuralgia.

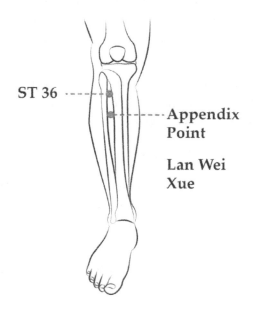

ST 36

Appendix
Point

Lan Wei
Xue

Lan Wei Xue – Appendix Point

The tender spot about 2 cun below ST 36, on the right leg only. This point will be tender when pressed, the most tender spot should be found for treatment.

Functions and Common Usage

Clears fire poison from the large intestine, treats chronic appendicitis, foot drop, and leg paralysis. Fire poison could be described as intense inflammation. This point specifically treats appendicitis, as well as it strongly improves circulation in the leg and foot to treat foot and leg problems.

Front of the Shoulder

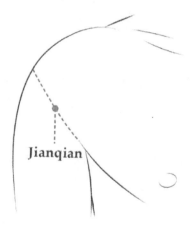

Jianqian

Jian Qian – Front of the Shoulder

Located on the front part of the shoulder joint, midway between the point LI 15 and the axillary crease. The axilla is the armpit.

Functions and Common Usage

This point treats pain and immobility of the shoulder joint.

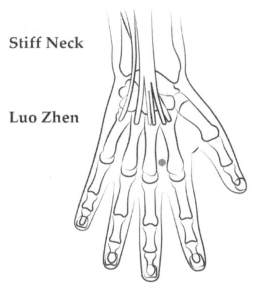

Luo Zhen – Stiff Neck Point
Located on the top of the hand, in the depression between the second and third hand bones.

Functions and Common Usage
Relieves stiff neck, neck pain, inability to turn your head to the side, and headache.

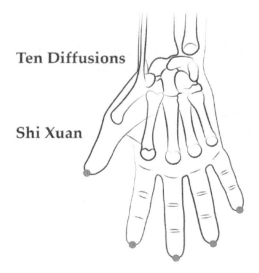

Shi Xuan – Ten Diffusions

On the tips of the ten fingers, about .1 cun from the fingernail.

Functions and Common Usage

Revive consciousness, and drain heat. Used for loss of consciousness, and stroke recovery.

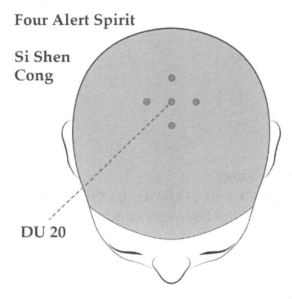

Si Shen Cong – Four Alert Spirit

A group of four points at the vertex of the head, each point is located one cun away from Du 20.

Functions and Common Usage

These points calm the spirit, and benefit the eyes and ears. These points can be used to stimulate your brain to improve memory, treat insomnia, dizziness, and eye problems.

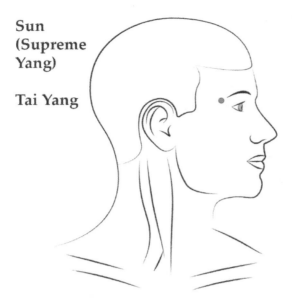

Sun
(Supreme
Yang)

Tai Yang

Tai Yang – Supreme Yang

In the depression about 1 cun posterior to the midpoint between the lateral end of the eyebrow and the outer canthus.

Functions and Common Usage

Reduces swelling, and relieves pain. Treats trigeminal neuralgia, eye disorders, vision problems, eye pain, and deviation of the mouth and eye.

Lift and Support

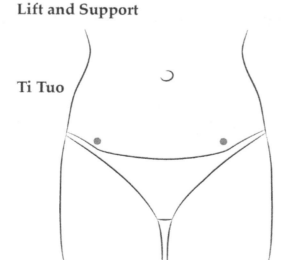

Ti Tuo

Ti Tuo – Lift and Support
Located 4 cun lateral to the midline, at the level of Ren 4, which is 3 cun below the navel.

Functions and Common Usage
This point is used for prolapse of the uterus, and painful menstruation. In many cases Chinese herbs are necessary to strengthen the body. Prolapse is caused by fatigue in most cases. Energy tonic herbs are given that restore energy levels.

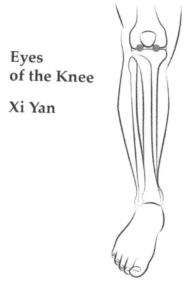

Eyes
of the Knee

Xi Yan

Xi Yan – Eyes of the Knee
Two points on either side of the patellar ligament. Located in the eyes of the knee, which are located by the kneecap.

Functions and Common Usage
Treats pain in the knee joint, difficulty moving the knee, and weak knees. This point is commonly combined with other points around the knee joint like He Ding, ST 34, ST 36, SP 9, and SP 10.

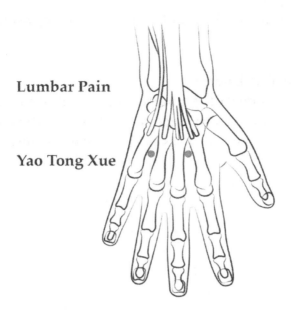

Lumbar Pain

Yao Tong Xue

Yao Tong Xue – Lumbar Pain Points

On the top of the hand, between the second and third hand bones, and between the fourth and fifth hand bones. There are two points on each hand.

Functions and Common Usage

Used for lower back pain.

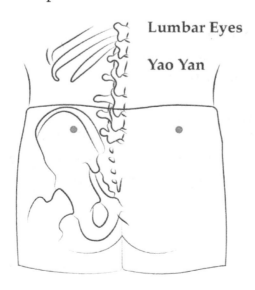

Lumbar Eyes

Yao Yan

Yao Yan – Lumbar Eyes
In the depression 3.5 cun lateral to the lower border of Lumbar vertebra 4.

Functions and Common Usage
Used to treat lower back pain, and strengthen the kidneys.

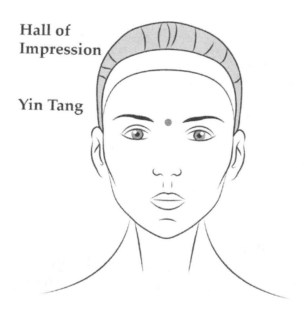

Hall of Impression

Yin Tang

Yin Tang – Hall of Impression, or Spirit Gate
Midway between the medial ends of the two eyebrows.

Functions and Common Usage
Calms the mind, benefits the nose, treats insomnia, and nasal congestion. This point is very effective to treat insomnia, and it is very calming.

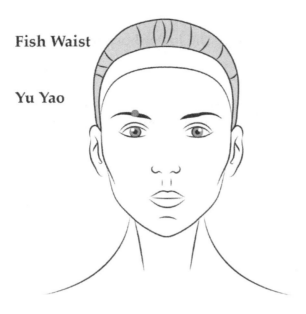

Yu Yao – Fish Waist
At the midpoint of the eyebrow.

Functions and Common Usage
Benefits the eyes. It can be used for eye pain, and drooping eyelids. Acupuncture is very effective to relax the tight muscles on the face that cause wrinkles.

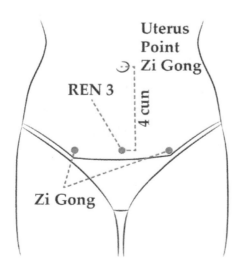

Zi Gong – Uterus Point, or Palace of the Child

Three cun lateral to Ren 3. Located 4 cun below the navel and 1 cun above the pubic bone.

Functions and Common Usage

Zi Gong regulates menstruation. It treats prolapse of the uterus, infertility, and abnormal uterine bleeding. This point is used a lot to treat infertility. It improves blood flow in the pelvis, and it has been shown to even unblock fallopian tubes in some cases.

How Acupuncture Improves Fertility

- Restores healthy blood flow in the pelvis
- Improve the Kidneys, which is how Chinese medicine treats hormonal imbalances
- Regulates the Liver, which regulates the hormones
- Restores complete health, which is necessary for healthy fertility

Acupuncture and Chinese herbal medicine should be given to both the male and female. Acupuncture restores health, it does not treat infertility as a separate entity. It restores health, so your body can function normally. Common patterns that are seen in infertility patients are:

- Liver Qi stagnation
- Kidney deficiency
- Blood stagnation

In addition to helping improve the odds of conception, acupuncture can also be used to improve the mother's health during pregnancy. If the mother gets acupuncture during her pregnancy, her baby is often very calm. The acupuncture treats and calms the baby, as it treats the mother. These babies are called *Acupuncture Babies*. It is a well-known phenomenon that *Acupuncture Babies* are very calm and cry less than other babies.

Resources

I used multiple sources for the images in this book. I cross-referenced several books and chose the most commonly used locations and functions of each point.

A Manual of Acupuncture by Peter Deadman, Mazin Al-Khafaji and Kevin Baker. This is the book acupuncture students use to learn point locations in school.

Acupuncture Points Images and Functions, by Arnie Lade. This book does not have all the points, and it does not have point images. It is an extremely good reference for a broad range of point functions.

Acupuncture A Comprehensive Text, Shanghai College of Traditional Medicine, by John O'Connor and Dan Bensky. This is called simply the "Shanghai Book" by most acupuncturists. It is a reference book for many acupuncture students.

The Foundations of Chinese Medicine by Giovanni Maciocia. This is the first year text for acupuncture students. It explains Chinese medicine diagnosis and Chinese medicine theory.

The Practice of Chinese Medicine by Giovanni Maciocia. This is the second year book for acupuncture students. Dozens of diseases are explained in Chinese medicine terms. It explains how to diagnose and treat diseases, which acupuncture points to use, and which herbal formulas to use.

Index

abdominal distension, 51, 142, 207, 208, 210
abdominal fullness, 214
abdominal pain, 55, 89, 90, 116, 117, 125, 165, 168, 169, 192, 194, 196, 197, 208, 209, 210, 214, 215, 217, 219
abscess, 172, 216, 219
acid reflux, 15, 18, 43, 159, 169, 170, 171, 172, 212
acupressure, 5, 7, 9, 11, 24, 25, 26, 27, 28, 29, 30, 75, 102, 103, 108, 123, 124, 128, 129, 139, 146, 151, 159, 196, 214, 237, 243
Acupuncture Babies, 253
Adjacent to Container of Fluids, 235, 244
allergic reactions, 239
allergies, 37, 123, 124, 127, 128, 151, 215, 228
amenorrhea, 188
An Mian, 235, 236
anemia, 188, 216
angina, 158
ankle pain, 58, 59, 61, 221
ankle sprain, 96
anxiety, 12, 15, 16, 33, 42, 103, 106, 158, 159, 170, 188
apathy, 14
appendicitis, 209, 215, 217
Appendix Point, 235, 245
arm atrophy, 126, 127
arm numbness, 127
arm pain, 12, 123, 126, 127, 129, 130, 178, 179, 180, 181, 229, 231
arm paralysis, 127
arrhythmia, 102, 103
Associated Point, 41, 42, 43, 44, 45, 46, 47
asthma, 16, 41, 54, 67, 107, 109, 111, 149, 151, 152, 181, 205, 206, 215, 219, 220, 240

Ba Feng, 235, 237, 238
Ba Xie, 235, 238
babies, breech, 62
back pain, 12, 45, 47, 48, 52, 54, 55, 57, 58, 59, 60, 61, 65, 75, 107, 177, 242
Back Shu, 41
belching, 18, 55, 56, 125, 186, 214
Bi Tong, 235, 239, 243
bile duct disorders, 239
bladder, 45, 46, 47, 110, 165, 166
bladder, regulates, 112
bleeding, 15, 116, 137, 186
blindness, color, 36, 79, 200
blindness, night, 43, 79, 84, 95
blindness, sudden, 36
blood deficiency, 18, 19, 188
blood pressure, high, 128, 139, 189, 216
blood, regulates, 191, 193
blood, stagnant, 43, 191
bloody stools, 186
bone aches, 14
bones, 40, 61, 95, 97, 104, 123, 138, 161, 186, 197, 206, 221, 222, 227, 246, 250
border of the red and white skin, 24
brain, 33, 71, 72, 86, 247
brain, clears, 68, 70, 109, 110, 161
breast, 18, 87, 156, 176, 206
breast abscess, 87, 176, 206
breast lumps, 18
breast pain, 87, 206
breath, bad, 15
breath, shortness, 148, 215, 220
breathing, difficult, 41, 54, 55, 110, 146, 152, 158, 172, 240
bronchitis, 16, 19, 40, 41, 54, 67, 148, 151, 206, 219
buttock pain, 91
calf pain, 58
Calm Difficult Breathing, 235, 240

255

cataracts, 36, 79, 95
cheek swelling, 82, 183
chest, 16, 40, 41, 42, 54, 67, 88, 100, 101, 118, 119, 146, 156, 158, 159, 170, 171, 172, 173, 180, 186, 198, 204, 205, 206
chest fullness, 88, 159, 205, 206
chest oppression, 186
chest pain, 41, 42, 100, 101, 118, 159, 170, 206
childbirth, 210
Chinese herbs, 12, 14, 17, 109, 113, 166, 167, 249, 256
Chinese medicine, 7, 8, 9, 11, 12, 13, 14, 15, 17, 18, 19, 94, 108, 110, 113, 138, 139, 165, 166, 177, 188, 208, 243, 253, 254
Chinese tonic herbs, 14, 167
coccyx, 48, 49, 64
cold, 14, 15, 16, 19, 40, 41, 68, 109, 122, 123, 127, 153, 157, 167, 215, 220
cold and flu, 16, 40, 41, 68, 122, 123, 124, 128, 151, 153, 215, 220
colic, 46
colitis, 209
collapsed Yang, 71
coma, 166
concentration, 71
conjunctivitis, 130, 177, 200
consciousness, loss, 176, 247
consciousness, revives, 71, 104, 122
constipation, 15, 27, 46, 109, 111, 116, 123, 127, 129, 196, 209, 210, 215, 220, 222, 228
constipation, severe, 229
convulsions, 59, 61, 137
cools heat, 156
cools the Blood, 189
Cordyceps, 14, 197
cornea, 80
cough, 16, 40, 41, 42, 54, 55, 67, 118, 119, 146, 149, 151, 152, 205, 220
coughing, 16, 41, 42, 67, 110, 149, 151, 157, 181, 206, 220, 240
coughing of blood, 157
coughing, stops, 151

cun, 22
cupping, 8, 193
Dan Nang Xue, 235, 239
deafness, 14, 45, 80, 81, 83, 107, 108, 123, 176, 177, 178, 184, 203, 226, 229, 232, 233, 234
deafness, sudden, 229, 230, 232
dementia, 109
depression, 18, 39, 59, 60, 61, 69, 81, 82, 83, 93, 97, 106, 107, 111, 113, 119, 123, 131, 138, 139, 140, 142, 146, 151, 152, 170, 173, 178, 180, 183, 184, 186, 187, 192, 202, 203, 213, 221, 227, 228, 230, 232, 234, 242, 246, 248, 251
deviation of the eye and mouth, 122, 183
deviation of the mouth, 133, 174, 201, 223, 244, 248
deviation of the mouth and eye, 174, 244, 248
diabetic neuropathy, 237
diaphragm, 42, 43, 55, 170
diaphragm spasms, 172, 215, 222
diaphragm, relaxes, 158
diarrhea, 45, 208, 209, 215, 217, 223
digestion, 11, 15, 44, 45, 56, 144, 167, 169, 187, 188, 198, 207, 216
digestion, improves, 45, 187
digestion, regulates, 56, 169, 187, 209
digestion, stagnant, 169
digestive issues, 43, 45, 116, 159
Ding Chuan, 235, 240
distal, 12
dizziness, 86, 137, 138, 188, 216, 220
dizziness from a Blood deficiency, 188
drug addiction, 31
ear acupuncture, 30, 34
ear blockage, 184, 227
ear discharge, 184
ear infections, 80, 123
ear inflammation, 184
ear pain, 226, 232, 234

ear, itching inside, 232
ear, swelling, 232
ears, 30, 45, 71, 98, 124, 182, 184, 226, 227, 228, 229, 230, 232, 233, 234, 247
ears, blocked, 86
ears, opens, 80, 176
eczema, 128, 189, 193
edema, 19, 45, 111, 112, 113, 187, 188, 190, 192, 208, 209, 215, 222
edema, pitting, 190
Eight Pathogens, 235, 238
Eight Winds, 235, 237
ejaculation, premature, 14, 210
elbow pain, 125, 126, 128, 129, 130, 177, 179, 232
emotions, 15, 109, 138
endocarditis, 42
endometriosis, 187
energy, 9, 13, 14, 15, 16, 17, 19, 28, 44, 45, 46, 71, 106, 108, 110, 124, 165, 166, 187, 197, 216, 226, 249
energy levels, 9, 14, 15, 16, 28, 44, 46, 110, 165, 166, 187, 216, 249
enteritis, 215, 217
epigastric pain, 169
epilepsy, 61, 67, 83, 177
Er Bai, 235, 241
esophageal constriction, 43, 172
eye disorders, 43, 95, 130, 248
eye disorders, all, 200
eye itching, 95
eye pain, 36, 39, 73, 79, 84, 85, 95, 179, 200, 234, 248, 252
eye pain, burning, 176
eye pain, bursting, 204
eye problems, 247
eye redness, 200, 234
eye swelling, 36
eye, inability to close, 201
eyelid spasm, 200
eyelid twitching, 183, 201, 204
eyelids, drooping, 252
eyes, 18, 36, 38, 39, 43, 45, 70, 79, 80, 84, 86, 95, 98, 124, 178, 179, 200, 204, 214, 227, 234, 247, 249, 252

eyes, dry, 79, 80, 226
eyes, itching, 200
eyes, red, 176
face, regulates, treats all face disorders, 124
facial paralysis, 122, 125, 174, 183, 201, 202, 203, 222, 223, 234, 244
fainting, 75
faints, 72
fallopian tubes, 253
farsightedness, 79
fatigue, 14, 15, 45, 107, 108, 109, 110, 165, 166, 187, 188, 197, 215, 216, 249
fatigue, chronic, 109
fear, 170
feet, heat in the soles, 218
fertility, 14, 253
fetus, calms, 108
fetus, inverted, 29
fetus, turning, 62
fever, 128, 156
finger pain, 177, 179
Fish Waist, 235, 252
flu, 16, 19, 68, 86, 123, 127, 148, 151, 216, 219, 220, 228
fluid retention, 112, 215, 222
flushed face, 16, 138
foot atrophy, 60, 222
foot drop, 96, 218, 221, 222
foot numbness, 237
foot pain, 97, 98, 112, 114, 188, 221, 222, 223, 237
foot paralysis, 188
foot sole, 60, 106
foot tendons, contraction of, 93
foot weakness, 96
foot, arch pain, 114
Four Alert Spirit, 235, 247
Four Gates, 124
Front of the Shoulder, 235, 245
Gallbladder, 5, 9, 24, 43, 55, 78, 79, 80, 81, 82, 83, 84, 85, 86, 87, 88, 89, 90, 91, 92, 93, 94, 95, 96, 97, 98, 140, 144, 235, 239
gallbladder inflammation, 96
Gallbladder Point, 235, 239

gallstones, 67, 239
gastritis, 15, 169, 170, 188, 215, 217, 220, 221
gastrocnemius muscle, 58, 93, 94, 114, 141
genital itching, 106
genital pain, 114, 137, 140, 189, 192, 210
genital pain and itching, 114
genital swelling, 136
getting the Qi, 27
glaucoma, 36, 79
Governing vessel, Du, 42, 64
gums, bleeding, 15
Hall of Impression, 235, 251
hallucinations, 157
hand pain, 123, 177
hand weakness, 178
He Ding, 212, 235, 241, 249
headache, 37, 38, 39, 83, 106, 122, 123, 125, 137, 177, 184, 189, 221, 226, 232, 246
headache due to ear issues, 184
headaches, 18, 59, 61, 62, 70, 82, 83, 85, 86, 97, 98, 123, 124, 125, 133, 139, 228, 237
headaches, occipital, 59, 177
hearing, 14, 45, 80
hearing loss, 80
heart attacks, 159
Heart Fire, 16, 42, 102, 104, 157, 158, 161
heart pain, 100, 102, 104, 158, 170
heart pounding, 102, 103, 158
heart rhythm, 102, 158
heart rhythm disorders, 158
heart, stabbing pain in, 102
heart, strengthens, 102, 159
heatstroke, 128
heel pain, 58, 59, 60, 107, 109, 110
hemiplegia, 61, 92
hemorrhoids, 46, 51, 58, 64, 65, 241
Hepatitis, 137, 139
hernia, 89, 137, 139, 140, 189, 209, 210
Herpes zoster, 128
hiatal hernia, 43, 159, 170

hiccups, 18, 55, 89, 149, 158, 169, 172
hip atrophy, 211
hip pain, 90, 91, 211
hives, 68, 92, 123, 124, 128, 156, 189, 193, 211, 216
hoarseness, 153
hormones, 13, 33, 139, 253
hormones, balances, 188
hot flashes, 109, 111
Hua Tuo's Paravertebral Points, 235, 242
hunger, 15
hypertension, 93, 137
hysteria, 157
immune system, 124, 128, 151, 215, 220
immune system tonic, 215
immune system, regulates, 124
immune system, strengthens, 68, 128
impotence, 189
incontinence, 14, 45, 47, 65, 107, 108, 112, 113, 164, 166, 189, 194, 197
incontinence, fecal, 196, 197
indigestion, 117, 126, 169, 187, 215, 217
infertility, 18, 19, 165, 166, 189, 210, 253
inflammation, 15, 17, 43, 47, 68, 125, 149, 153, 169, 170, 193, 215, 217, 239, 245
inguinal hernia, 136
insomnia, 12, 14, 15, 16, 18, 26, 27, 33, 42, 71, 103, 104, 106, 107, 108, 111, 112, 137, 139, 158, 159, 161, 189, 236, 247, 251
intercostal neuralgia, 41
intestinal abscess, 209, 215, 217
intestinal obstruction, 209, 217
intestines, 46, 129, 196, 209, 215, 217, 222, 229
intestines, moistens, 196
intestines, opens, 228

intestines, regulates, 46, 116, 126, 168, 196, 197, 209, 217, 219, 220, 223
irritability, 18, 104, 137, 138
itching, 28, 42, 92, 128, 193, 200, 232
itching anywhere, 193
jaundice, 43, 55, 67, 137, 139, 140, 178, 188
jaw, 80, 81, 124, 183, 202, 203, 243
jaw clenching, 202, 203
jaw dislocation, 203
jaw pain, 80, 243
jawbone, 82, 184, 203
Jia Bi, 235, 243
Jia Cheng Jiang, 235
Jian Qian, 235, 245
joint deformity, 40
Kidney deficiency, 45, 189, 253
kidney dialysis, 108
kidney disorders, 65
kidney stones, 45, 108, 166, 210
Kidney Yang, 14, 107
kidneys, strengthens, 45, 65, 89, 106, 110, 111, 112, 114, 165, 166
knee osteoarthritis, 212
knee pain, 51, 93, 94, 114, 141, 193, 211, 212, 213, 242
knee weakness, 107
knee, eyes of, 235, 249
kneecap, 193, 211, 212, 213, 214, 219, 249
labor induction, 59, 189
labor, expedites, 111
labor, induces, 87, 124
labor, speeds, 62
LAc, Licensed Acupuncturist, 3, 7
lactation, 97, 216
lactation, insufficient, 87, 180, 198, 206
lactation, promotes, 172, 176
lactation, regulates, 158
Lan Wei Xue, 235, 245
large intestine, regulates and moistens, 127
Lasik dry eye, 79
lateral malleolus, 24

leg atrophy, 51, 65, 91
leg pain, 59, 96, 211, 212, 216, 217
leg weakness, 96, 216, 217
leukorrhea, 210, 216
Lift and Support, 235, 249
lips and cheeks swelling, 201
lips, stiff, 76
Liver Fire, 18, 19, 137, 138
Liver Yang, 138, 139
Liver, regulates, 55, 95, 96, 97, 136, 189, 253
lockjaw, 75, 174, 202, 203, 223, 232
lower back pain, 14, 46, 47, 48, 51, 57, 58, 59, 60, 61, 64, 65, 66, 75, 91, 96, 109, 110, 112, 165, 210, 211, 212, 219, 250, 251
lower back pain referring to the genitals, 219
lower leg atrophy, 95, 213
lower leg pain, 95, 218, 219, 220, 221
Lower leg paralysis, 59
Lumbar Eyes, 235, 251
Lumbar Pain Point, 235, 250
lung function, 148, 220
lungs, regulates, 41, 124, 128, 147, 149, 172, 173
lungs, strengthens, 146, 151, 215
Luo Zhen, 235, 246
magnetic pellets, 25, 104, 139, 159, 160
Magrain Ion pellets, 30, 31
mania, 104, 110, 114, 157
manic depression, 103, 114, 177, 208
manic psychosis, 208
mastitis, 89, 118, 172, 176, 206
medial malleolus, 24
memory, 14, 16, 71, 73, 103, 104, 107, 158, 247
memory, improves, 72
menstrual, 19, 140, 191, 209, 210
menstrual cramps, 191
menstrual pain, 209
menstruation, 18, 110, 111, 113, 139, 142, 166, 167, 188, 193, 210, 253

menstruation, irregular, 110, 115, 116, 136

menstruation, painful, 110, 249

menstruation, regulates, 89, 142, 187, 189, 209, 210

migraines, 17, 19, 78, 86, 95, 97, 98, 139

mind, calms, 33, 42, 61, 67, 68, 70, 71, 73, 75, 83, 100, 102, 103, 104, 109, 111, 124, 158, 170, 177, 188, 208, 219, 251

morning sickness, 158, 159, 187

mouth deviation, 133

mouth, difficulty opening, 202

mouth, dry, 14, 16, 109, 112

Moxa, 167

moxibustion, 62, 167

MSOM, 3, 8

mucus, 16, 17, 19, 41, 149, 151, 152, 219, 220

mucus in the lungs, 16, 41, 152, 220

mugwort, 62, 167

muscle spasms, 93

muscle tension, 139

muscle weakness, 18

NADA ear protocol, 31

nails, brittle, 18

nasal congestion, 251

nasal discharge, 72

nasal obstructions, 72

nasal polyps, 73, 133, 239

nausea, 9, 18, 26, 45, 117, 158, 159

nausea during pregnancy, 158

navel pain, 209

nearsightedness, 36, 73, 85, 200

neck pain, 59, 67, 69, 86, 87, 95, 96, 174, 177, 178, 246

neck stiffness, 39, 61, 68, 85, 123, 179

neck, stiff, 40, 61, 179, 181, 246

nephritis, 45, 65, 112, 113, 210

night sweats, 14, 16

nose, 38, 39, 73, 74, 75, 84, 124, 239, 243, 251

nose, runny, 75

nosebleeds, 75, 76, 102, 124, 133, 137

occiput pain, 97

optic nerve atrophy, 36, 43, 79, 95

palpitations, 15, 16, 41, 42, 102, 103, 104, 110, 158, 159, 171

pancreatitis, 43, 144, 209, 215

paralysis, 47, 201, 211, 216, 219, 220, 245

passes out, 72

Peaceful Sleep, 235, 236

Penetrating the Nose, or Nose Passage, 235

pericarditis, 42, 171

peritonitis, 46

Phlegm Heat, 16, 17, 177

Phlegm Point, 17, 19, 220

pleurisy, 40, 41

pneumonia, 40, 41, 220

pregnancy, 9, 59, 87, 111, 124, 189, 209, 253

pregnancy, points contraindicated, 9

prolapse, 71, 215, 249

prostatitis, 47

psoriasis, 42, 128

pulse, 13

rashes, 128

rectal prolapse, 46, 64, 72, 166, 241

rectum, 71, 166

relaxing, 33, 40, 106, 139

restless fetus disorder, 139

retinal hemorrhage, 79

rib pain, 41, 89, 93, 96, 98, 100, 239

roundworms, 201

sacrum, 32, 46, 48, 57, 65, 91, 177

sacrum pain, 60

scapula pain, 180, 181

sciatica, 51, 60, 91, 92, 93

Sea of Blood, 193

seizures, 60, 61, 75, 137

Shi Xuan, 235, 247

shoulder, 19, 54, 55, 87, 100, 126, 130, 131, 179, 180, 181, 218, 227, 231, 232, 245

shoulder pain, 19, 54, 86, 87, 100, 126, 128, 130, 131, 177, 180, 181, 218

shoulder stiffness, 128

Si Shen Cong, 235, 247
sighing, 18, 138
sinus blockage, 38, 71, 73, 243
sinus congestion, 37, 38, 39, 41, 62, 73, 84, 85, 124, 133, 239
sinus headaches, 72, 133, 201, 239, 243
sinus inflammation, 73, 201
Sinus Point, 235
sinus pressure, 133
sinuses, 38, 133, 151, 239, 243
sinuses, inflamed, 38
sinuses, opens, 37, 41, 71, 72, 75, 133, 201, 243
skin diseases, 42, 128, 189
skin disorders, inflammatory, 128
sleeping too much, 111
small intestines, 165
smell, inability, 133
smell, sense of, 38, 133
speech, loss of after a stroke, 86
spinal nerves, regulate, 242
spine, 32, 40, 47, 64, 87, 90, 131, 180, 211, 242
spine stiffness, 40, 47
spine, regulates, 75, 177
startled easily, 16
Stiff Neck, 177, 235, 246
Stiff Neck Point, 177, 246
Stomach Fire, 15, 169, 170, 220, 221
stomach pain, 15, 45, 207, 208, 212, 215
stomach, calms, 158
stomach, regulates, 117, 126, 158, 220, 222
stress, 9, 12, 17, 18, 31, 33, 86, 94, 138, 139, 189, 203
stroke, 75, 127, 129, 130, 157, 158, 162, 166, 167, 176, 183, 202, 237, 247
stroke recovery, 130, 157, 247
stroke, inability to speak after, 69
stuttering, 102
Supreme Yang, 235, 248
swallowing, difficulty, 18, 55, 110, 170, 172, 182, 204, 215, 216
sweating, night, 102, 112

sweating, regulates, 112, 124
Tai Yang, 235, 248
tailbone, 32, 46, 48, 49, 57, 65
tear production, excess, 200, 201, 204
teeth grinding, 203
Ten Diffusions, 235, 247
tendons, 40, 52, 61, 93, 94, 95, 124, 151, 157, 158, 161, 221
tendons, relaxes, 51, 60, 93, 174, 227
testicles, 113
thigh pain, 92, 212
thirst, 14, 15, 16, 18
throat pain, 122, 220, 226, 228
throat, burning pain, 169
throat, dry, 112, 153
throat, moistens, 111, 173, 176, 182, 204
throat, sore, 111, 122, 123, 124, 125, 128, 153, 202, 205
Ti Tuo, 235, 249
tinnitus, 14, 18, 45, 70, 80, 81, 83, 107, 108, 125, 138, 176, 177, 178, 184, 203, 226, 227, 228, 229, 230, 232, 233, 234
TMJ, 80, 202, 203
toe pain, 97, 187, 222
tongue, 13, 16, 69, 102, 173, 188, 226
tongue stiffness, 69, 102, 188
tongue, pain at the root, 226
tonsillitis, 122, 123, 125
toothache, 81, 122, 123, 124, 126, 178, 183, 201, 202, 203, 223, 230, 233
trigeminal neuralgia, 122, 123, 133, 183, 200, 201, 203, 223, 244, 248
tuberculosis, 54, 68
Tui Na, 8
Two Whites, 235, 241
ulcers, 169
urinary disorders, 115, 164
urinary retention, 166
urinary, painful urinary dysfunction, 47
urinate, inability to, 57, 64, 164, 189

urination, 14, 45, 57, 107, 108, 112, 166, 189, 194, 210
urination, difficult, 46, 57, 115, 164, 166, 210
urination, dribbling, 111
urination, frequent, 107, 110, 111, 112
urination, painful, 110, 113, 189, 194, 210
urination, urgent, 107
urine retention, 64, 189, 210
uterine bleeding, abnormal, 113, 136, 167, 191, 253
uterine prolapse, 72, 90, 106, 110, 111, 113, 115, 139, 142, 166, 189, 210
uterus, 71, 142, 143, 165, 166, 191, 210, 249, 253
Uterus Point, also called the Palace of the Child, 235
uterus, regulates, 165, 166, 191
vaginal itching, 167
vertigo, 38, 60, 83, 98, 139, 184
vertigo due to ear problems, 184
vision, 84, 95, 248
vision problems, 139, 248
vision, blurred, 18, 36, 38, 43, 45, 61, 70, 72, 86, 95, 110, 138, 179, 188, 204, 216, 232, 234
vision, dimness of, 232
voice, 132
voice, benefits, 228
voice, loss of, 153, 229
voice, sudden loss, 101, 102, 182, 228, 230
voice, weak, 16
vomiting, 15, 18, 43, 55, 102, 117, 139, 158, 169, 170, 186, 187, 207, 208, 209, 215
vomiting blood, 102
waking at night to urinate, 108
weak legs, 14, 212
wheezing, 17, 108, 119, 146, 148, 151, 152, 172, 206, 220, 240
whiplash, 39, 177
whooping cough, 41, 67, 220
willpower, 110

wrinkles, 252
wrist, 21, 101, 102, 103, 124, 149, 151, 152, 157, 158, 159, 160, 161, 178, 227, 228, 229, 230, 241
wrist contracture, 178
wrist pain, 96, 124, 227
Xi Yan, 235, 249
Yang, 13, 14, 72, 165, 166
Yao Tong Xue, 235, 250
Yao Yan, 235, 251
Yin, 13, 14, 16, 41, 166, 189, 235, 251
Yin Tang, 235, 251
Yu Yao, 235, 252
Zi Gong, 235, 253

About the Author

Deborah Bleecker is a Licensed Acupuncturist, and has a Master of Science degree in Oriental Medicine. A degree in Oriental Medicine is a combination of acupuncture, and Chinese herbal medicine. This is a complete system of medicine that has been used for thousands of years.

She was injured on the job in 1994 and lived with chronic pain until she decided she would have to find her own answers to her health problems. Medical doctors told her that her pain was incurable, but she was able to recover with the help of acupuncture and Chinese herbs.

She can be reached at deborahbleecker@gmail.com.

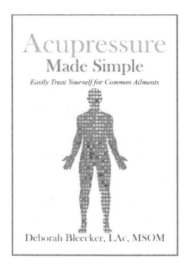

If you ever wanted to help yourself with effective and easy to find acupressure points, this book was written for you. I have chosen the most powerful acupressure points, and made them easy to find, and easy to understand.

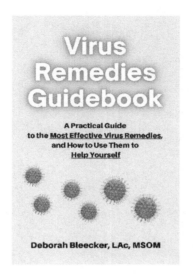

Viruses are everywhere. They cause colds and flu, and many other deadly diseases. Although most people are unaware of it, there are many herbs that have been used for hundreds of years, and have also been proven by modern science to reduce viral replication. It does not matter what type of virus it is, there are natural solutions available over the counter.

These herbal remedies are:
- Easy to use
- Easy to find
- Used for hundreds of years
- Backed by modern scientific research

This book will show you how to help yourself. You don't need to suffer, if you take the right supplements.

Made in United States
Orlando, FL
06 February 2024

43307497R00148